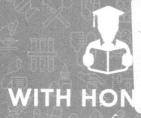

WITH HON...

Pre-Clinical
MEDICINE

MCQs and EMQs with Detailed Solutions

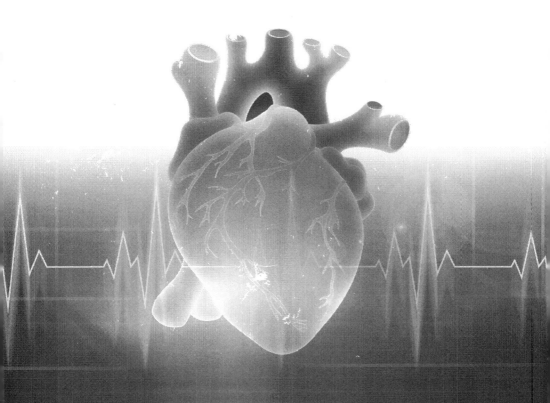

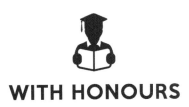

WITH HONOURS

Website: withhonours.co.uk
Email: contact@withhonours.co.uk

© 2018 With Honours. All rights reserved.

No part of this book may be reprinted, reproduced, transmitted, or utilised in any form by any electronic, mechanical, or other means, now known or hereafter invented, including photocopying, microfilming, and recording, or in any information storage or retrieval system, without permission in writing from the publisher.

First edition 2018

ISBN: 978-1-9999452-3-7

Cover design by Alessandro Migliorato, Milano

Interior design by Danijela Mijailovic

Notices

As new research findings come to light, and our appreciation and understanding of the medical sciences evolves, changes in drug therapy, medical devices and proper treatment may be required. The publisher has made every effort to ensure that the information given in this book is accurate and up to date at the time of publication.

The publisher does not assume and hereby disclaims any liability to any party for results obtained from the use of information contained herein and any loss, damage, or disruption caused by errors or omissions, whether such errors or omissions result from accident, negligence, or any other cause.

CONTENTS

	Preface	5
1	Cell and Tissue Biology (MCQs)	7
2	Proteins (MCQs)	27
3	Enzymes and Metabolism (MCQs)	43
4	Clinical Genetics (MCQs)	61
5	Embryology and Reproduction (MCQs)	79
6	The Respiratory System (MCQs)	97
7	The Cardiovascular System (MCQs)	115
8	The Gastrointestinal System (MCQs)	133
9	The Renal System (MCQs)	151
10	Haematology (MCQs)	169
11	Endocrinology (MCQs)	187
12	The Immune System (MCQs)	205
13	Microbiology and Infection (MCQs)	223
14	The Musculoskeletal System (MCQs)	241
15	The Nervous System (MCQs)	257
16	Public Health (EMQs)	277
17	Pharmacology and Therapeutics I (EMQs)	289

18	Pharmacology and Therapeutics II (EMQs)	301
19	Pharmacology and Therapeutics III (EMQs)	313
20	Clinical Biochemistry (EMQs)	325
21	Clinical Interpretation (EMQs)	337
	Answer Key	349

Preface

The aim of this book is to equip you with the medical knowledge and clinical acumen necessary to excel in your pre-clinical exams. Success at medical school demands an in-depth understanding of fundamental scientific principles, as well as the ability to integrate and apply this knowledge in different clinical contexts. Each chapter of this book has been rigorously developed in order to help you do just that, with over 500 practice questions in total. Detailed and informative solutions are also provided at the end of each chapter, enabling you to constructively engage with the material in a methodical and systematic manner.

This book consists of 21 chapters, which each cover a particular aspect of the pre-clinical medical course, from embryology and reproduction to public health. For clarity and ease of use, each chapter will follow the same format: 24 multiple choice questions (MCQs) or extended matching questions (EMQs) on a given topic, with answers and detailed solutions to each question at the end of the chapter. These practice questions can be completed under exam conditions (for which we would advise a 30-minute time frame per chapter) or attempted sequentially to help consolidate your learning. Comprehensive and informative solutions are provided to help you not only identify the correct responses, but outline why other answers would not be appropriate. We have also carefully designed each chapter in order to help accommodate targeted and effective revision. You may find that you score very highly in one topic, for example haematology, but poorly in another, such as clinical biochemistry. If this is the case, you can take advantage of the self-contained nature of each chapter and modify your revision accordingly. Along these lines, there is no need to work through the chapters chronologically; you are free to start with subject areas in which you are particularly confident, before moving to weaker areas and vice versa.

A clinical focus is sustained throughout the book in order to help develop nascent clinical reasoning skills, alongside confidence and competence in the medical sciences. The more clinically-orientated questions are particularly useful as they provide you with an opportunity to contextualise your growing medical knowledge; an invaluable skill for the clinical years of medical school. Given the specialist nature of some of these questions, additional contextual information will be provided, where necessary, in order to facilitate interaction with the subject matter.

In keeping with the subject knowledge requirements of the undergraduate medical curriculum, the questions are set at a level equivalent to that expected of a first and second year undergraduate medical student. A difficulty rating has also been assigned to each question (Easy, Moderate or Hard), in order to help you gauge your performance, and pinpoint particular strengths and areas for improvement. We have purposefully ordered questions of varying difficulty (8 easy, 8 moderate and 8 hard) throughout each chapter, with easy ones seamlessly integrated with those classified as moderate and hard. It is important to note that the questions marked as 'hard' have been written with the most ambitious students in mind. These questions have been included to stretch your appreciation and understanding of the subject matter and, as such, may challenge the limits of your knowledge.

The following table provides a useful indicator of performance:

Score for each chapter	Descriptor
<8	Further Revision Needed
8 -11	Satisfactory Performance - review areas of weakness
12 -15	Good Performance - identify specific gaps in knowledge
16 -19	Very Strong Performance - consolidate knowledge
20+	Exceptional (on the road to graduating **With Honours!**)

We wish you every success in your pre-clinical exams and your future medical career,

The **With Honours** team

CHAPTER 1
Cell and Tissue Biology (MCQs)

1.1. There are five levels of structural organisation within the human body. These levels are ordered, with increasing complexity, as follows:

A) Tissues, cells, organs, organ systems, organism
B) Organs, organ systems, cells, tissues, organism
C) Cells, tissues, organs, organ systems, organism
D) Organ systems, cells, tissues, organs, organism

1.2. Cell death can be divided into two types: apoptosis (programmed cell death) and necrosis (abnormal, unintended cell death). Which of the following statements is **true** with regard to the differences between apoptosis and necrotic cell death?

A) Necrosis is an active process that requires energy
B) Apoptosis is a passive process, which does not expend energy
C) Apoptosis takes place in response to physiological or pathological signals, while necrosis occurs in response to cell injury
D) Apoptosis incites an inflammatory reaction and the release of harmful products

1.3. There are several distinct morphological types of necrosis: coagulative, caseous, colliquative and gangrenous (wet and dry). Colliquative (liquefactive) necrosis is characteristic of which of the following?

A) Tuberculosis (TB)
B) Myocardial infarction (MI)
C) Bowel infarct
D) Brain injury due to haemorrhage

1.4. Which of the following statements is **false** with regard to the differences between prokaryotic and eukaryotic cells?

A) Eukaryotes contain a well-defined membrane bound nucleus, as well as other membrane bound organelles (such as mitochondria)
B) Prokaryotes lack a membrane bound nucleus
C) Eukaryotic ribosomes are smaller than prokaryotic ribosomes
D) Prokaryotic genes lack introns

1.5. The skin is composed of three major layers: an outermost epidermis, middle dermis and inner subcutis. Which of these layers does **not** contain any blood vessels?

- A) Epidermis
- B) Dermis
- C) Subcutis
- D) All of the above

1.6. The epidermis of thick skin contains five layers: stratum basale, stratum spinosum, stratum granulosum, stratum lucidum and stratum corneum. In contrast, the epidermis of thin skin only contains four layers. Which of the following cellular layers is **not** found in thin skin?

- A) Stratum basale
- B) Stratum spinosum
- C) Stratum lucidum
- D) Stratum corneum

1.7. Which of the following statements is **true** with regard to the common characteristics of epithelial tissue?

- A) Epithelial tissue is innervated but avascular (contains no blood vessels) and therefore dependent on diffusion from underlying capillary beds
- B) Epithelia are attached to an underlying basement membrane and exhibit polarity
- C) Epithelia are characterised by cellularity and have a strong regenerative ability
- D) All of the above

The following **two** questions concern epithelial nomenclature.

1.8. Epithelia are categorised based on prevailing cellular features. These include shape and number of cell layers, as well as various specialisations. An epithelia that is several layers thick and consists of flattened cells would be described as a:

A) Simple squamous epithelium
B) Stratified squamous epithelium
C) Pseudostratified columnar epithelium
D) Transitional cuboidal epithelium

1.9. Epithelia can also be categorised based on mitotic activity, function and numerous specialisations. An epithelia that contains tall cells, cilia and appears stratified but is not as all of the cells make direct contact with the underlying basement membrane would be described as a:

A) Ciliated pseudostratified columnar epithelium
B) Keratinised simple squamous epithelium
C) Secretory stratified cuboidal epithelium
D) Proliferative transitional squamous epithelium

1.10. Connective tissue is composed of two basic elements: an extracellular matrix (ECM) and various different cell types (including fibroblasts, adipocytes and immune cells). Which of these various cell types is associated with the synthesis of collagen, elastin and glycosaminoglycans (GAGs)?

A) Adipocytes
B) Fibroblasts
C) Immune cells
D) None of the above

1.11. Cartilage is classified into three types: hyaline, elastic and fibrocartilage. Hyaline cartilage is the most abundant of the three types, and is predominantly found in which of the following locations?

A) Trachea and the soft part of the nose
B) Cartilaginous portions of the ears
C) Intervertebral discs
D) Pubic symphysis

1.12. Which of the following cellular transport mechanisms requires energy from the hydrolysis of adenosine triphosphate (ATP)?

A) Diffusion
B) Facilitated Diffusion
C) Osmosis
D) Active Transport

1.13. The nucleus is surrounded by a nuclear envelope, which consists of _____ cellular membrane(s).

A) One
B) Two
C) Three
D) Four

1.14. Which of the following organelles has a mildly acidic internal pH and contains degradative enzymes (collectively known as acid hydrolases)?

A) Smooth endoplasmic reticulum (SER)
B) Rough endoplasmic reticulum (RER)
C) Lysosomes
D) Golgi apparatus

1.15. Biological membranes are selectively permeable barriers. Accordingly, a pure lipid bilayer will only be freely permeable to water, small gases, small hydrophobic molecules and small uncharged polar molecules. Which of the following molecules is **not** able to pass freely through a phospholipid bilayer?

A) Carbon dioxide
B) Ethanol
C) Amino acids
D) Oxygen

CHAPTER 1: Cell and Tissue Biology (MCQs)

1.16. There are three major types of cell population found in adult tissue: labile, stable and permanent. Which of the following types of cell population is found in the liver?

A) Stable (quiescent)
B) Labile
C) Permanent
D) None of the above

1.17. Labile cell populations are found in:

A) Kidney tubules
B) Epithelia
C) Neurones
D) Muscle

1.18. Which of the following terms **best** describes the healing process, if injured tissue is replaced by fibrosis and scarring and specialised function is lost?

A) Repair
B) Regeneration
C) A and B
D) None of the above

1.19. Wound healing can be divided into three types: first (primary) intention, second (secondary) intention and third intention or delayed primary closure. Which of the following characteristics is associated with healing by **second** intention?

A) Wounds with minimal tissue loss, such as a clean, uninfected surgical wound
B) Skin edges apposed, for instance with sutures or staples
C) Extensive scarring and granulation tissue
D) Good haemostasis

1.20. Acute inflammation is the initial tissue reaction to injury or infection. Which of the following processes is **not** a major component of acute inflammation?

A) Changes in vessel calibre (after an initial period of transient vasoconstriction, vasodilation occurs)
B) Decreased vascular permeability
C) Fluid exudate formation
D) Cellular exudate formation

1.21. Which of the following statements is **false** with regard to the differences between acute and chronic inflammation?

A) Acute inflammation is short-lived and takes place over hours to days, while chronic inflammation is of prolonged duration and can last weeks, months, or years
B) Chronic inflammation mainly involves innate immunity, while acute inflammation is associated with innate and adaptive immunity
C) The cells that play a key role in acute inflammation are neutrophils, mast cells and macrophages, while macrophages, lymphocytes and plasma cells are the main cellular components in chronic inflammation
D) Amyloidosis, cachexia and anaemia of chronic disease are clinical features of chronic inflammation

1.22. There are five cardinal features of acute inflammation. These include: redness (rubor), heat (calor), swelling (tumor), pain (dolor) and _____.

A) Myalgia
B) Rhinitis
C) Rigors
D) Loss of function

1.23. There are a number of cancer-specific characteristics that can be used to differentiate between neoplastic and normal cells. Which of the following is **not** a hallmark of cancer cells?

A) Independence from positive growth factors and resistance to negative growth factors
B) Loss of contact inhibited cell division, resistance to apoptosis and immortality
C) Invasion, metastasis and angiogenesis
D) Genomic stability

1.24. Benign epithelial and mesenchymal tumours usually end in the suffix -oma. Which of the following terms is used to describe a benign tumour of surface (non-glandular or non-secretory) epithelium?

A) Adenoma
B) Papilloma
C) Osteoma
D) Lipoma

CHAPTER 1

Cell and Tissue Biology (MCQs)

Answers and Detailed Solutions

The difficulty rating for each question (Easy, Moderate or Hard) can be found in parentheses next to the correct answer.

1.1. C (Easy)

The five levels of structural organisation within the human body are ordered, with increasing complexity, as follows: cells, tissues, organs, organ systems, organism. Cells are the structural and functional units of life. Cells that are similar in structure and function aggregate to form tissues, such as muscle and connective tissue. In turn, several tissues that work together to perform a specific function are known as an organ. Likewise, an organ system is a group of organs that work together to perform one or more particular functions. Finally, various organ systems integrate to form a functioning organism.

1.2. C (Moderate)

Apoptosis (programmed cell death) is an active process that requires energy. In contrast, necrosis (abnormal, unintended cell death) is a passive process that does not expend energy. Apoptosis takes place in health and disease, in response to physiological (such as embryogenesis) or pathological (such as viral infection) signals. Conversely, necrosis occurs in response to cell injury. Accordingly, necrosis incites an inflammatory reaction and the release of harmful products, while apoptosis does not release any harmful products.

1.3. D (Hard)

Neural tissue has very little supporting stroma and liquefies upon cell death, usually leaving a cyst. Accordingly, colliquative (liquefactive) necrosis is most likely to be seen in a brain injury due to haemorrhage. Caseous or 'cheese-like' necrosis is characteristic of tuberculosis (TB), while wet gangrene is likely to develop following a bowel infarct, due to the action of superimposed bacterial infection. Coagulative necrosis is the most common type of necrosis, and is typically seen in myocardial tissue following a myocardial infarction (MI).

1.4. C (Easy)

Prokaryotes (derived from Greek roots meaning 'before the nucleus') lack a membrane bound nucleus. Conversely, eukaryotes (derived from Greek roots meaning 'true nucleus') contain a well-defined membrane bound nucleus, as well as other membrane bound organelles (such as mitochondria). Prokaryotic ribosomes are smaller than eukaryotic ribosomes. In addition, while eukaryotic genes may have introns, prokaryotic genes do not.

1.5. A (Easy)

The epidermis does not contain any blood vessels and, as such, is dependent on the underlying dermis for its nourishment. The epidermis is a continuously proliferating keratinised stratified squamous epithelium, which lies in direct contact with the external environment. The dermis provides structural and metabolic support to the epidermis, and is rich in nerve fibres, lymphatics, blood vessels and sensory receptors. The subcutis is deep to the dermis, and consists of loose connective tissue with variable amounts of adipose tissue.

1.6. C (Hard)

The stratum lucidum (skin of the sole) is absent in thin skin. Along these lines, the epidermis of thin skin consists of the following four cellular layers: stratum basale (the basal layer), stratum spinosum (the prickle cell layer), stratum granulosum (the granular layer) and stratum corneum (the keratin layer).

1.7. D (Moderate)

Epithelial tissue is innervated but avascular (contains no blood vessels) and therefore dependent on diffusion from underlying capillary beds. Epithelia are attached to an underlying basement membrane and described as polar, as they possess apical and basal surfaces. Likewise, epithelia are characterised by cellularity, as their cells are tightly bound to one another. In addition, epithelia undergo germinative cell division and are thus characterised by a strong regenerative ability.

1.8. B (Hard)

Epithelia are classified based on shape: squamous (flattened cells), cuboidal (cube-shaped cells stacked next to one another) and columnar (tall cells, typically with a basal nucleus). Epithelia are also classified based on the number of cell layers: simple (one layer), stratified (several layers thick), pseudostratified (appear stratified but are not, as all of the cells make direct contact with the underlying basement membrane), and transitional (stratified, but the appearance of the cells and layers changes as it stretches or relaxes). The epithelia described in this question would thus be called a stratified squamous epithelium.

1.9. A (Hard)

Epithelia are categorised based on mitotic activity, function and numerous specialisations: ciliated (if it contains cilia), keratinised (if it contains keratin), secretory (if it has cytoplasmic secretary vacuoles) and proliferative (if it is composed of mitotic figures). The epithelia described in this question would thus be called a ciliated pseudostratified columnar epithelium.

1.10. B (Moderate)

Fibroblasts synthesise collagen and elastin (fibres that run within the extracellular matrix), as well as glycosaminoglycans (GAGs). Conversely, adipocytes store fat and immune cells such as white blood cells (leukocytes) help to fight infection. For further information about the different types of immune cells found within the human body refer to the detailed solutions for questions 12.3., 12.6., 12.20. and 12.22. in chapter 12.

1.11. A (Easy)

Hyaline cartilage is found in the soft part of the nose and the trachea, where rings of hyaline cartilage provide structural support to help keep the airway open. Elastic cartilage is found in a limited number of locations, such as the cartilaginous portions of the ears. Fibrocartilage is a very tough material found in the intervertebral discs and the pubic symphysis.

1.12. D (Easy)

Diffusion, facilitated diffusion and osmosis are all passive (do not require energy) cellular transport mechanisms as they occur along a concentration gradient. Active transport, however, requires energy from the hydrolysis of adenosine triphosphate (ATP), as it involves moving a substance against its concentration gradient.

1.13. B (Easy)

The nucleus is surrounded by a nuclear envelope, which consists of two cellular membranes; an inner and outer nuclear membrane. These two membranes fuse at nuclear pores, and this allows large molecules such as RNA and complexes such as ribosomes (which are assembled in the nucleolus) to pass between the nucleus and the cytosol in a highly regulated manner.

1.14. C (Moderate)

Lysosomes have a mildly acidic internal pH and contain numerous degradative enzymes (collectively known as acid hydrolases). These enzymes degrade extracellular macromolecules brought into the cell and delivered to lysosomes via the endocytotic pathway, as well as cellular components that have become obsolete. Tay-Sachs disease (TSD) is an autosomal recessive neurodegenerative disorder, caused by a mutation and subsequent deficiency of the lysosomal enzyme, hexosaminidase A (HEX A). The endoplasmic reticulum (ER) is an interconnected network of closed, flattened membrane-bound sacs known as cisternae. The smooth endoplasmic reticulum (SER) does not contain any ribosomes, and is the site of fatty acid and phospholipid biosynthesis. The rough endoplasmic reticulum (RER) is covered with ribosomes, which are responsible for protein synthesis. Proteins synthesised in the rough endoplasmic reticulum are then transported in vesicles to the Golgi apparatus or Golgi complex. The Golgi apparatus consists of a series of flattened membrane-bound sacs, involved in protein modification and translocation.

1.15. C (Easy)

Small Gases (such as oxygen and carbon dioxide) and small uncharged polar molecules (such as ethanol), can freely pass through the phospholipid bilayer. In contrast, charged polar molecules (such as amino acids), large polar molecules (such as glucose) and charged molecules (such as ions) are not able to freely cross the membrane.

1.16. A (Moderate)

Stable (quiescent) cell populations are found in the liver (and the kidney tubules). These cells have a good regenerative capacity, and although they have a low physiological turnover, if necessary cell turnover can be vastly increased.

1.17. B (Moderate)

Labile cell populations are found in epithelia. Epithelial tissue has a high cell turnover and an excellent regenerative capacity, owing to the presence of an active stem cell population. Permanent cell populations are found in neurones and muscle. These cells have no physiological turnover and, as such, do not possess any regenerative capacity. Stable (quiescent) cell populations are found in the kidney tubules (and the liver).

1.18. A (Moderate)

Healing is comprised of two processes: repair and regeneration. Healing by repair describes a situation in which injured tissue is replaced by fibrosis and scarring and specialised function is concomitantly lost. Healing by regeneration occurs when injured tissue is replaced by tissue of the same type, and specialised function returns to normal.

1.19. C (Hard)

Healing by first (primary) intention occurs in wounds with minimal tissue loss, such as a clean, uninfected surgical wound. These wounds will have good haemostasis, and the skin edges will be apposed, for instance with sutures or staples. Healing by second (secondary) intention occurs in wounds with extensive tissue loss. Accordingly, the wound edges cannot be apposed. This can be attributed to the degree of tissue loss, or because apposition is not physically possible. In addition, there may be an infection, large haematoma or the presence of an obstructive foreign body. Healing by second intention is not a fundamentally different process to healing by primary intention, but involves more granulation tissue and extensive scarring. Healing by third intention or delayed primary closure, occurs when the wound is left open to heal for a few days prior to closure, this technique is often employed for wounds that are significantly contaminated.

1.20. B (Hard)

Acute inflammation is a rapid host response which delivers white cells (such as the neutrophil polymorph) and plasma proteins (such as antibodies) to the site of infection or injury. The vessels undergo changes to facilitate this process. There are changes in vessel calibre (after an initial period of transient vasoconstriction, vasodilation occurs). This is mediated by the effects of histamine and nitric oxide (NO) on vascular smooth muscle, and is accompanied by an increase (not a decrease) in vascular permeability. This increased permeability results in the escape of protein rich fluid into tissue from the vessels, and the formation of fluid exudate. The loss of fluid into tissues and increased calibre of vessels, also results in slower blood flow and increases the thickness (viscosity) of the blood, leading to stasis and the formation of cellular exudate. Accordingly, neutrophils move towards the vascular endothelium and stick to it (in a process referred to as margination or pavementing) and then migrate through the wall into tissues. Exudate can be defined as extravascular fluid with a high protein content, which contains cellular debris.

1.21. B (Moderate)

Acute inflammation is short-lived and takes place over hours to days, while chronic inflammation is of prolonged duration and can last weeks, months, or years. Acute inflammation mainly involves innate immunity, while chronic inflammation is associated with innate and adaptive immunity. The cells that play a key role in acute inflammation are neutrophils, mast cells and macrophages, while macrophages, lymphocytes and plasma cells are the main cellular components in chronic inflammation. Amyloidosis, cachexia and anaemia of chronic disease are clinical features of chronic inflammation. Amyloid is a protein produced in response to chronic inflammation, which forms sheets and deposits in different tissues around the body. Patients lose a lot of weight and are cachexic, as the body uses up a lot of its energy supplies in ongoing chronic inflammation. Furthermore, the cytokines produced have an impact upon the kidneys and bone marrow, which affects the production of red blood cells (erythropoiesis), leading to anaemia of chronic disease.

1.22. D (Easy)

The five cardinal features of acute inflammation include: redness (rubor), heat (calor), swelling (tumor), pain (dolor) and loss of function (functio laesa). Myalgia (muscle pain), rigors and rhinitis may be associated with acute inflammation, but are not specifically included in the five classical signs of acute inflammation.

1.23. D (Hard)

Tumour cells acquire the ability to grow in the absence of positive growth factors, and resist the action of negative growth factors. Normal cells deteriorate with age and have a finite replicative life span. Conversely, tumour cells can be distinguished by the loss of contact inhibited cell division, resistance to apoptosis and immortality. Cancer cells can also invade local tissues (invasion) and migrate from their site of origin to secondary sites (metastasis). Similarly, they are able to stimulate the development of new blood vessels (angiogenesis). In addition, genomic instability (not stability) is a distinguishing hallmark of cancer cells.

1.24. B (Hard)

Benign epithelial tumours usually end in the suffix -oma. Along these lines, a benign tumour of surface (non-glandular or non-secretory) epithelium is known as a papilloma and a benign tumour of glandular or secretory epithelium is called an adenoma. Likewise, benign mesenchymal tumours often have the suffix -oma. Osteoma refers to a benign tumour of bone, and lipoma describes a benign tumour of adipose tissue.

CHAPTER 2
Proteins (MCQs)

2.1. All α-amino acids have a common structure. Each consists of a central carbon atom (α-carbon) to which four different chemical groups are attached. Which of the following chemical groups is **not** part of this general structure?

A) Amino Group
B) Carboxyl Group
C) Alkene Group
D) Hydrogen atom

2.2. Proteins are linear polymers of amino acids covalently linked to one another via peptide (or amide) bonds. Which of the following statements is **false** with regard to peptide (or amide) bonds?

A) They are formed between the carboxyl group of one amino acid and the side chain or R-group of the subsequent amino acid in the polypeptide chain
B) They exhibit partial double-bond characteristics
C) They are formed by a condensation reaction (the loss of a water molecule)
D) They are broken apart by a hydrolysis reaction (the addition of a water molecule)

2.3. The α-helix and β-pleated sheet are examples of which level of protein structural organization?

A) Primary structure
B) Secondary structure
C) Tertiary structure
D) Quaternary structure

2.4. Protein structure is stabilised by a number of different types of forces and interactions, both covalent and non-covalent in character. Which of the following is an example of a **covalent** interaction?

A) Van der Waals forces
B) Disulphide bridges
C) Electrostatic attraction
D) None of the above

2.5. The secondary structure of a protein is stabilised by which of the following interactions?

  A) Disulphide bridges
  B) Hydrogen bonds
  C) Ionic bonds
  D) Van der Waals forces

2.6. The unique chemical properties of each α-amino acid are determined by their respective side chain or R-group. Which of the following α-amino acids contains a **polar** side chain?

  A) Serine (Ser)
  B) Leucine (Leu)
  C) Alanine (Ala)
  D) Valine (Val)

2.7. Which of the following α-amino acids contains **sulphur**?

  A) Histidine (His)
  B) Phenylalanine (Phe)
  C) Cysteine (Cys)
  D) Tyrosine (Tyr)

2.8. Which of the following α-amino acids is **aliphatic**?

  A) Tyrosine (Tyr)
  B) Tryptophan (Trp)
  C) Alanine (Ala)
  D) Phenylalanine (Phe)

2.9. Which of the following α-amino acids is **non-polar** and **aromatic**?

  A) Phenylalanine (Phe)
  B) Glutamine (Gln)
  C) Threonine (Thr)
  D) Asparagine (Asn)

2.10. All α-amino acids display optical isomerism **except**:

A) Methionine (Met)
B) Cysteine (Cys)
C) Glycine (Gly)
D) Phenylalanine (Phe)

2.11. Which of the following statements is **false** with regard to α-amino acids?

A) Those found in proteins are all L-amino acids
B) They are amphoteric
C) At neutral pH Lysine (Lys) is basic (positively charged)
D) At neutral pH Arginine (Arg) is acidic (negatively charged)

2.12. Mutations leading to amino acid substitution can be classified as either conservative or non-conservative. Which of the following is a **conservative** substitution?

A) Alanine (Ala) > Isoleucine (Ile)
B) Leucine (Leu) > Lysine (Lys)
C) Arginine (Arg) > Tryptophan (Trp)
D) Valine (Val) > Glutamate (Glu)

2.13. The interior of water-soluble proteins consists of hydrophobic amino acid residues, while the exterior of these proteins predominantly contains hydrophilic amino acid residues. Which of the following residues is most likely to be found in the **interior** of water-soluble proteins?

A) Valine (Val)
B) Aspartate (Asp)
C) Glutamate (Glu)
D) Lysine (Lys)

2.14. Which of the following proteopathies is **not** a prion-related illness?

A) Alzheimer's disease (AD)
B) Scrapie
C) Bovine Spongiform Encephalopathy (BSE)
D) Creutzfeldt-Jakob disease (CJD)

2.15. Which of the following statements is **false** with regard to prion proteins and the infections they typically cause?

A) They contain genetic material (nucleic acids)
B) New variant Creutzfeldt-Jakob disease (nvCJD) is associated with the ingestion of infected beef
C) Human prion diseases can be sporadic
D) Prion diseases can be inherited via genetic defects or transmitted when contaminated brain or spinal cord matter gets into the human food chain

2.16. Which of the following statements is **true** with regard to the biosynthesis of collagen?

A) Synthesis takes place, in part, within fibroblasts and partly within the extracellular spaces of connective tissue
B) Peptidase enzymes cleave extension peptides from procollagen in order to form tropocollagen
C) Intramolecular and intermolecular covalent cross linking of tropocollagen helps to give collagen its structural strength and rigidity
D) All of the above

2.17. The enzymes prolyl hydroxylase and lysyl hydroxylase are responsible for the hydroxylation of Proline (Pro) and Lysine (Lys) residues during collagen biosynthesis. Which of the following co-factors is required for the successful functioning of these enzymes?

A) Folic acid (vitamin B_9)
B) Biotin (vitamin B_7)
C) Ascorbic acid (vitamin C)
D) Thiamine (vitamin B_1)

2.18. The primary structure of collagen is largely composed of a repeating triplet of amino acids. Which of the following residues is found in the **highest** proportion in this repetitive sequence?

A) Proline (Pro)
B) Glycine (Gly)
C) Hydroxyproline (HyP)
D) Hydroxylysine (HyL)

2.19. Osteogenesis imperfecta (OI) or 'brittle bone disease' is a heterogenous group of inherited disorders, characterised by bone fragility and increased fracture risk, and predominantly caused by mutations in type I collagen. Which is of the following is the most serious form of the disease?

A) Type I
B) Type II
C) Type III
D) Type IV

2.20. Dupuytren's contracture (Dupuytren's disease) is a potentially disabling connective tissue disorder caused by excessive collagen synthesis. Which of the following enzymes is used in the clinical treatment of Dupuytren's contracture?

A) Trypsin
B) Collagenase
C) Angiotensin-converting enzyme (ACE)
D) Amylase

2.21. There are nine essential amino acids (EAA). Which of the following statements is **false** with regard to these essential amino acids?

A) They cannot be synthesised by the human body
B) They cannot be obtained from an individual's diet
C) Methionine (Met) is an essential amino acid
D) Phenylalanine (Phe) is an essential amino acid

2.22. Which of the following is an α-**imino** acid?

A) Proline (Pro)
B) Cysteine (Cys)
C) Glutamate (Glu)
D) Serine (Ser)

2.23. Which of the following amino acids are **both** glucogenic and ketogenic?

- A) Leucine (Leu) and Lysine (Lys)
- B) Tyrosine (Tyr) and Tryptophan (Trp)
- C) Glycine (Gly) and Histidine (His)
- D) Alanine (Ala) and Serine (Ser)

2.24. The clinical manifestations of scurvy result from malformation in which of the following structural proteins?

- A) Actin
- B) Collagen
- C) Elastin
- D) Fibrillin

CHAPTER 2

Proteins (MCQs)

Answers and Detailed Solutions

The difficulty rating for each question (Easy, Moderate or Hard) can be found in parentheses next to the correct answer.

2.1. C (Easy)

Each α-amino acid consists of a central carbon atom (α-carbon) to which four different chemical groups are attached: a hydrogen atom, amino group, carboxyl group and a variable side chain or R-group.

2.2. A (Moderate)

Peptide (or amide) bonds are formed between the carboxyl group of one amino acid and the amino group of the subsequent amino acid in the polypeptide chain. They exhibit partial double-bond characteristics and, as such, display considerably less rotational freedom than a single covalent bond. In addition, peptide bonds are formed by a condensation reaction (the loss of a water molecule) and broken apart by a hydrolysis reaction (the addition of a water molecule).

2.3. B (Easy)

The α-helix and β-pleated sheet are two of the most commonly encountered forms of secondary protein structure. They are stabilised by interchain and/or intrachain hydrogen bonds, and constitute the local spatial arrangement of amino acid residues in the polypeptide chain. The primary protein structure refers to the linear amino acid sequence. Likewise, the tertiary structure refers to the folding and coiling of the primary and secondary structures into a compact, three-dimensional shape. Quaternary structure refers to the arrangement in space of the different polypeptide chains (sub-units) within a protein. Hydrogen bonds, Van der Waals forces, disulphide bridges, electrostatic attraction and the hydrophobic effect, all help to stabilise the tertiary and quaternary structure of proteins.

2.4. B (Hard)

Van der Waals interactions are non-covalent, weak forces of attraction that occur between electrically neutral molecules. Likewise, electrostatic attraction is non-covalent in character, and occurs between oppositely charged side chains or R-groups. In contrast, disulphide bridges are covalent links that form between Cysteine (Cys) residues. Each of these interactions helps to stabilise the tertiary and quaternary structure of proteins.

2.5. B (Easy)

The secondary structure of a protein is stabilised by hydrogen bonds between the carbonyl group (C=O) of one peptide (or amide) bond and the amino group (N-H) of another peptide bond. These interactions can be interchain (between different amino acid chains) and/or intrachain (between two parts of the same chain). Disulphide bridges, ionic bonds and Van der Waals forces all help to stabilise the tertiary and quaternary structure of proteins.

2.6. A (Moderate)

Alanine (Ala), Leucine (Leu) and Valine (Val) all contain non-polar side chains. In contrast, Serine (Ser) contains a polar side chain. The classification of α-amino acids is based on the different chemical properties of their respective side chains or R-groups.

2.7. C (Easy)

Cysteine (Cys), along with Methionine (Met), contains sulphur. This allows cysteine residues to form disulphide bridges, which help to stabilise the tertiary and quaternary structure of proteins.

2.8. C (Moderate)

Tyrosine (Tyr), Tryptophan (Trp) and Phenylalanine (Phe) are aromatic, as they each contain a ring structure(s), and are hydrophobic in nature. In contrast, Alanine (Ala) is aliphatic as it does not contain any ring structures.

2.9. A (Moderate)

Glutamine (Gln), Threonine (Thr) and Asparagine (Asn) all contain polar side chains or R-groups. In contrast, Phenylalanine (Phe) contains a non-polar side chain and is aromatic.

2.10. C (Moderate)

Methionine (Met), Cysteine (Cys) and Phenylalanine (Phe) exhibit optical activity, as they each consist of four different chemical groups arranged tetrahedrally around a chiral or asymmetric carbon. Glycine (Gly), on the other hand, is an achiral molecule which does not display optical isomerism. This is because the side chain or R-group of glycine is a hydrogen atom and, as such, the molecule has two identical groups (hydrogen atoms) attached to its central carbon atom (α-carbon).

2.11. D (Hard)

At neutral pH, Lysine (Lys) and Arginine (Arg) are basic (positively charged). In like manner, α-amino acids are amphoteric, as they are able to act as both a proton donor (acid) and a proton acceptor (base). In addition, the α-amino acids found in proteins are all L-amino acids or L-isomers, as they rotate the plane of plane-polarised light in a counterclockwise manner (i.e. are levorotatory).

2.12. A (Hard)

Mutations leading to amino acid substitution can be classified as either conservative or non-conservative, based on the biochemical properties of the residues involved. Conservative mutations result from the substitution of an amino acid with similar biochemical properties to the original residue, and lead to the formation of a normal polypeptide variant. In contrast, non-conservative mutations involve the substitution of a biochemically different amino acid residue. These mutations are much more likely to be disease-causing than conservative substitutions. The substitution of Alanine (Ala) for Isoleucine (Ile) is a conservative mutation seen in haemoglobin, as both residues are non-polar and, as such, the hydrophobic interior of the molecule is maintained. In contrast, the substitution of hydrophobic Leucine (Leu) for the electrically charged (basic) Lysine (Lys) is a non-conservative change. Likewise, substitution of the large, aromatic and non-polar residue, Tryptophan (Trp) for the electrically charged (basic) Arginine (Arg) is a non-conservative mutation. Similarly, the replacement of hydrophobic Valine (Val) for the negatively charged (acidic) Glutamate (Glu) is a non-conservative substitution.

2.13. A (Hard)

Valine (Val) is non-polar and, as such, is likely to be found in the interior hydrophobic region of water-soluble proteins. In contrast, Aspartate (Asp), Glutamate (Glu) and Lysine (Lys) are electrically charged residues, and are thus likely to be found in the exterior portion of water-soluble proteins.

2.14. A (Easy)

Prions are the causative agents in bovine spongiform encephalopathy (BSE) or mad cow disease, scrapie and Creutzfeldt-Jakob disease (CJD). In contrast, Alzheimer's disease (AD) is an amyloid-related illness.

2.15. A (Moderate)

Prions can be set apart from viruses by the fact that they do not contain genetic material (nucleic acids). In addition, new variant Creutzfeldt-Jakob disease (nvCJD) is associated with the ingestion of infected beef. Human prion diseases can be sporadic (as showcased in sporadic Creutzfeldt-Jakob disease) or inherited via genetic defects. Similarly, prion diseases are often transmitted when contaminated brain or spinal cord matter gets into the human food chain. For example, Kuru used to be present among the Fore people of Papa New Guinea due to ritual cannibalism, as it was customary practice for the brain tissue of deceased relatives to be ingested by fellow family members.

2.16. D (Moderate)

The biosynthesis of collagen is a multistep process, which results in the formation of a triple helix, composed of three polypeptide chains. The first stages take place within fibroblasts and the final stages occur within the extracellular spaces of connective tissue. Peptidase enzymes cleave extension peptides from procollagen in order to form tropocollagen. In

CHAPTER 2: Proteins (MCQs)

addition, intramolecular and intermolecular covalent cross linking of tropocollagen helps to give collagen its structural strength and rigidity.

2.17. C (Moderate)

The enzymes prolyl hydroxylase and lysyl hydroxylase require the co-factor ascorbic acid (vitamin C) in order to successfully hydroxylate Proline (Pro) and Lysine (Lys) amino acid residues during collagen biosynthesis. Hydroxyproline (HyP) helps to stabilise the collagen triple helix through the formation of hydrogen bonds. In like manner, Hydroxylysine (HyL) residues are glycosylated and involved in the formation of covalent cross-links between collagen chains. Collagen is thus structurally weakened in ascorbic acid deficiency.

2.18. B (Hard)

The primary structure of collagen is largely composed of the following repeating triplet of amino acids:

$$(Gly - X - Y)_n$$

X is often Proline (Pro), and Y is often Hydroxyproline (HyP). Glycine (Gly) occurs every third residue, and thus constitutes 33% of the total amino acid residues in collagen. This is because glycine is the smallest amino acid residue and, as such, it can occupy positions at the centre of the collagen triple helix.

2.19. B (Hard)

The clinical severity of osteogenesis imperfecta (OI) or 'brittle bone disease' fluctuates depending upon the nature of the mutation. Type II is the most serve form of the disease. Infants with type II OI rarely survive birth due to significant skeletal deformity. Type III is the most serious form with which people survive, and often marked by short stature in adulthood. Type IV is milder than types II and III, but more severe than type I. Along these lines, type I is the mildest and most frequent form of the disease.

2.20. B (Easy)

The enzyme collagenase (a member of the matrix metalloproteinase family of zinc containing enzymes) breaks down collagen and, as such, can be employed in the clinical treatment of Dupuytren's contracture (Dupuytren's disease).

2.21. B (Easy)

The majority of the twenty naturally occurring α-amino acids can be synthesised in the human body, however, there are nine that cannot. These include: Methionine (Met), Histidine (His), Phenylalanine (Phe), Isoleucine (Ile), Leucine (Leu), Lysine (Lys), Threonine (Thr), Tryptophan (Trp) and Valine (Val). These nine essential amino acids need to be obtained from an individual's diet.

2.22. A (Hard)

Cysteine (Cys), Glutamate (Glu) and Serine (Ser) are all α-amino acids. In contrast, Proline (Pro) is not an α-amino acid, but an α-imino acid as it contains a secondary amino group.

2.23. B (Hard)

Amino acids that are glucogenic can be converted to glucose via gluconeogenesis. In contrast, ketogenic amino acids can be used to produce ketone bodies. Glycine (Gly), Histidine (His), Alanine (Ala) and Serine (Ser) are all glucogenic, while Leucine (Leu) and Lysine (Lys) are purely ketogenic. Tyrosine (Tyr) and Tryptophan (Trp) are both ketogenic and glucogenic and, as such, give rise to glucose and ketone bodies.

2.24. B (Easy)

The clinical manifestations of scurvy can be attributed to the abnormal synthesis of the structural protein collagen. This connective tissue disorder is caused by a deficiency in ascorbic acid (vitamin C), which is necessary for the hydroxylation of Proline (Pro) and Lysine (Lys) residues during collagen biosynthesis. For further information about the critical role played by ascorbic acid in collagen biosynthesis refer to the detailed solution for question 2.17. in this chapter.

CHAPTER 3
Enzymes and Metabolism (MCQs)

3.1. Which of the following statements is **false** with regard to enzyme function?

A) Enzymes are biological catalysts
B) Enzymes shift the position of equilibrium
C) Enzymes increase the rate at which equilibrium is reached
D) Enzymes lower the activation energy of a reaction

3.2. The rate of an enzyme-catalysed reaction is affected by:

A) Temperature
B) pH
C) Substrate concentration
D) All of the above

The following **three** questions concern the mechanisms behind reversible and non-reversible enzyme inhibition.

3.3. Which of the following statements is **true** with regard to reversible **competitive** enzyme inhibition?

A) Inhibition is overcome by a low substrate concentration
B) Inhibition is overcome by a high substrate concentration
C) Inhibition is not affected by a low substrate concentration
D) Inhibition is not affected by a high substrate concentration

3.4. Which of the following statements is **true** with regard to reversible **non-competitive** enzyme inhibition?

A) Inhibition is not affected by a high substrate concentration
B) Inhibition is affected by a high substrate concentration
C) Inhibition is affected by a low substrate concentration
D) Substrate and inhibitor simultaneously bind to the enzyme's active site

3.5. Which of the following statements is **false** with regard to **irreversible** enzyme inhibition?

A) Aspirin is a competitive irreversible enzyme inhibitor
B) Ibuprofen is a competitive irreversible enzyme inhibitor
C) It occurs via the covalent modification of amino acid side chains in the enzyme's active site
D) Irreversible inhibition can be competitive or non-competitive

3.6. Glucose-6-phosphate dehydrogenase (GP6D) deficiency is seen in which of the following disorders?

A) Favism
B) Phenylketonuria (PKU)
C) Ehlers-Danlos syndrome (EDS)
D) Lesch-Nyhan syndrome (LNS)

3.7. Which of the following models can be used to explain how an enzyme binds to its substrate?

A) The lock-and-key model
B) The induced-fit model
C) A and B
D) None of the above

3.8. The active site of the proteolytic enzyme trypsin is composed of three critical amino acid residues. Which of the following residues is **not** found in the active site of this digestive enzyme?

A) Histidine (His)
B) Glycine (Gly)
C) Aspartate (Asp)
D) Serine (Ser)

3.9. Which of the following proteins is **not** a serine protease?

A) Chymotrypsin
B) Trypsin
C) Antithrombin
D) Elastase

The following **five** questions concern the Michaelis-Menten equation and the Lineweaver-Burk plot.

The Michaelis-Menten equation measures the rate of an enzyme-catalysed reaction as a function of substrate concentration:

$$V = \frac{V_{max}[S]}{[S] + K_m}$$

3.10. Which of the following statements is **false** with regard to the different variables (V, [S]) and parameters (V_{max}, K_m) employed within the Michaelis-Menten equation?

A) V refers to the velocity of the reaction
B) [S] refers to the substrate concentration
C) V_{max} refers to the theoretical maximum rate of enzyme catalysis
D) V_{max} can be measured directly

3.11. The Michaelis constant (K_m) refers to:

A) The substrate concentration at which the reaction rate (V) is equal to its theoretical maximum value
B) The substrate concentration at which the reaction rate (V) is one-quarter of its theoretical maximum value
C) The substrate concentration at which the reaction rate (V) is half its theoretical maximum value
D) The substrate concentration at which the reaction rate (V) is double its theoretical maximum value

3.12. The Michaelis constant (K_m) reflects the affinity of an enzyme for its substrate. Which of the following statements is **true** with regard to the value of K_m?

A) A numerically low K_m indicates high affinity
B) A numerically high K_m indicates low affinity
C) A numerically high K_m indicates high affinity
D) A and B

The Lineweaver-Burk plot (LB plot) is an experimentally determined derivation of the Michaelis-Menton equation. This double reciprocal plot can be used to estimate V_{max} and K_m, and to characterise the effects of competitive and non-competitive inhibition on enzyme activity.

3.13. Which of the following statements is **true** with regard to the effects of **competitive** inhibition on the Lineweaver-Burk plot?

A) K_m is unchanged
B) K_m is decreased
C) V_{max} is unchanged
D) V_{max} is increased

3.14. Which of the following statements is **true** with regard to the effects of **non-competitive** inhibition on the Lineweaver-Burk plot?

A) V_{max} is unchanged
B) V_{max} is increased
C) K_m is decreased
D) K_m is unchanged

3.15. Raised serum enzyme levels can provide a reliable indicator of tissue damage and disease. Which of the following is **not** associated with an increase in serum enzyme activity?

A) Increased synthesis, including cellular proliferation
B) Cell death and cell membrane damage
C) Defective or unexpectedly slow clearance
D) Inborn errors of metabolism (IEM)

3.16. The clinical measurement of enzyme activity in serum can be of diagnostic value in a great many conditions. Elevated serum amylase is most likely to be seen in which of the following conditions?

A) Prostatic carcinoma
B) Acute myocardial infarction (AMI)
C) Liver disease
D) Acute pancreatitis

3.17. Deficiency in which of the following enzymes is linked to the pathogenesis of pulmonary emphysema?

A) Alpha-1-antitrypsin (AAT)
B) Chymotrypsin
C) Trypsin
D) Elastase

3.18. Glycolysis is tightly controlled by a number of different enzymatic steps. Which of the following glycolytic enzymes is involved in the conversion of glucose to glucose-6-phosphate?

A) Pyruvate kinase
B) Hexokinase
C) Phosphofructokinase
D) Glycogen phosphorylase

3.19. Which of the following statements is **true** with regard to glycolysis?

A) Occurs in the cytosol of all cells
B) Adenosine triphosphate (ATP) is synthesised under aerobic and anaerobic conditions in this pathway
C) Glucagon inhibits the pathway
D) All of the above

3.20. The mitochondrial matrix enzyme pyruvate dehydrogenase (PDH) catalyses the conversion of pyruvate to acetyl CoA in the link reaction. The pyruvate dehydrogenase complex is **activated** in which of the following situations?

A) When energy levels are high
B) When pyruvate dehydrogenase is in its dephosphorylated form
C) When pyruvate dehydrogenase is in its phosphorylated form
D) When there is a high cellular ratio of NADH:NAD$^+$

3.21. Which of the following is **not** a key regulatory enzyme in the Krebs cycle (tricarboxylic acid cycle)?

A) Glycogen synthase
B) Citrate synthase
C) Isocitrate dehydrogenase
D) α-ketoglutarate dehydrogenase

3.22. Which of the following statements is **false** with regard to the Krebs cycle (tricarboxylic acid cycle)?

A) Occurs in the mitochondrial matrix
B) The reduced coenzymes NADH and FADH$_2$ are generated
C) The cycle is inhibited by a low ATP: ADP ratio
D) Carbon dioxide is released as a waste product

3.23. Cyanide inhibits complex ___ of the electron transport chain.

A) I
B) II
C) III
D) IV

3.24. Which of the following statements is **false** with regard to the electron transport chain (respiratory chain)?

A) As electrons are transferred between complexes free energy is released
B) Electrons donated by NADH enter through complex I
C) Electrons donated by $FADH_2$ enter through complex II
D) Complexes I, II, III and IV pump protons (H^+) out of the mitochondrial matrix and across the inner mitochondrial membrane into the intermembrane space

CHAPTER 3
Enzymes and Metabolism (MCQs)

Answers and Detailed Solutions

The difficulty rating for each question (Easy, Moderate or Hard) can be found in parentheses next to the correct answer.

3.1. B (Easy)

Enzymes are proteins (with the exception of catalytic RNAs), which function as biological catalysts. As such, they serve to speed up the rate of metabolic reactions without being altered themselves. Enzymes increase the speed at which equilibrium is reached but do not shift the position of equilibrium within a chemical reaction. Accordingly, the presence of an enzyme significantly lowers the activation energy needed for a given reaction to proceed.

3.2. D (Easy)

The rate of an enzyme-catalysed reaction can be affected by temperature, pH and substrate concentration. As substrate concentration is increased, the rate of reaction increases in a linear fashion until it reaches a 'saturation' point. This occurs when all the enzyme binding sites are occupied by substrate molecules. Once this plateau has been reached, higher substrate concentration has very little influence on enzyme activity. In addition, every enzyme has an optimum temperature and pH. Enzymes in the human body have evolved to exhibit maximal catalytic activity at physiological temperature and pH (roughly 37°C and 7.4 respectively). There are, of course, exceptions to this rule. Lysosomal enzymes have evolved to possess optimal catalytic activity around pH 5. This is an important protective mechanism as if these hydrolytic enzymes were to leak out of cells, their release would lead to cellular autolysis, were it not for the fact that they lose enzymatic activity at cytoplasmic pH. Similarly, the digestive enzyme pepsin is adapted to the acidic environment of the stomach, with a pH optimum around 2.

3.3. B (Hard)

Competitive inhibition is dependant upon the relative concentrations of inhibitor and substrate in a reaction and, as such, is overcome by a high substrate concentration. This is because the substrate is able to out-compete the inhibitor and bind to the enzyme's active site. During competitive inhibition substrate and inhibitor molecules contend to bind to the enzyme's active site, therefore, if you raise substrate concentration the inhibitor will be displaced from the enzyme's active site. This is competitive as opposed to non-competitive inhibition, as both inhibitor and substrate molecules can attach to the enzyme's active site, but cannot do so simultaneously.

3.4. A (Moderate)

Non-competitive enzyme inhibition is not affected by a high substrate concentration, as the inhibitor molecule binds at a site distinct from the enzyme's active site. Accordingly, substrate molecules cannot out-compete non-competitive inhibitors, as they are both binding to different sites.

3.5. B (Hard)

Irreversible enzyme inhibition occurs via the covalent modification of amino acid side chains in the enzyme's active site. In a similar vein to reversible enzyme inhibition, irreversible inhibition can be either competitive or non-competitive in nature. Aspirin is a competitive irreversible inhibitor, which covalently modifies the serine residue in the active site of cyclooxygenase-1 (COX-1) and cyclooxygenase-2 (COX-2). In contrast, ibuprofen is a competitive reversible inhibitor, which non-covalently modifies cyclooxygenase (COX).

3.6. A (Moderate)

Favism is caused by a deficiency in the cytoplasmic enzyme, glucose-6-phosphate dehydrogenase (GP6D). Phenylketonuria (PKU) is caused by deficiency in the enzyme phenylalanine hydroxylase, which converts Phenylalanine (Phe) to Tyrosine (Tyr). Similarly, Ehlers-Danlos syndrome (EDS) refers to a group of inherited, clinically heterogeneous connective tissue disorders, linked to mutations in the genes responsible for collagen synthesis. Lesch-Nyhan syndrome (LNS) is linked to a deficiency in the enzyme, hypoxanthine-guanine phosphoribosyltransferase (HGPRT).

3.7. C (Easy)

Two different models have been put forward to explain how an enzyme binds to its substrate: the lock-and-key model (Fischer template hypothesis or rigid template model) and the induced-fit model. The former was proposed towards the end of the nineteenth century, and describes enzymatic catalysis in terms of enzyme-substrate complementarity. This model likens enzyme-substrate interaction to the way a key fits into a lock. According to this mechanism, the enzyme and substrate each possess a fixed and rigid geometrical conformation and, as such, fit exactly into one another. This helps to explain why enzymes will often only bind to specific substrates. Such a theory, however, cannot be uncritically applied to all enzyme-catalysed reactions. Accordingly, the induced-fit model was proposed in the middle of the twentieth century. This is a modified version of the lock-and-key model, and proposes that the enzyme undergoes a conformational change once it has bound to its substrate in order to complete the fit. In reality, the enzyme-substrate relationship can be described in terms of both complementarity (the lock-and-key model) and conformational change (the induced-fit model). To this end, both models help contribute to our understanding of how an enzyme binds to its substrate.

3.8. B (Easy)

Glycine (Gly) is not found in the active site of trypsin. Therefore, the active site of this digestive enzyme contains the catalytic triad of Serine (Ser), Histidine (His) and Aspartate (Asp).

3.9. C (Easy)

The proteolytic, digestive enzymes chymotrypsin, trypsin and elastase are all serine proteases. As such, each of these protein-cleaving enzymes contains a reactive serine amino acid residue in their active site. The considerable parallels in sequence and structure between these enzymes has led many to postulate that they evolved from a common precursor, by the process of divergent evolution. In contrast, antithrombin is a serpin or serine protease inhibitor, which inactivates thrombin (coagulation factor IIa) and coagulation factors in the intrinsic and extrinsic coagulation pathways, including IXa, Xa, XIa, and XIIa. For further information about the coagulation factors and the coagulation cascade refer to the detailed solutions for questions 10.12., 10.13., 10.15., 10.17. and 10.18. in chapter 10.

3.10. D (Easy)

V_{max} refers to the theoretical maximum rate of enzyme catalysis, attainable at substrate saturation level. As such, it is a theoretical value and cannot be measured directly. The rate of an enzyme-catalysed reaction is called V, the velocity of the reaction. Likewise, [S] refers to substrate concentration.

3.11. C (Moderate)

The Michaelis constant (K_m) is a kinetic constant, which refers to the substrate concentration ([S]) at which the reaction rate (V) is half its theoretical maximum value (V_{max}).

3.12. D (Hard)

A numerically low K_m value for an enzyme indicates that it has a high affinity for its substrate. This is because only a low concentration of substrate is required to saturate the enzyme. To this end, a numerically high K_m value for an enzyme indicates that it has a low affinity for its substrate.

3.13. C (Hard)

In the Lineweaver-Burk plot, the y-intercept is equivalent to $1/V_{max}$, the x-intercept corresponds to $-1/K_m$ and the slope equals K_m/V_{max}. The slope and intercept values of a plot can thus be deployed to determine the kinetic parameters, V_{max} (the theoretical maximum rate of reaction) and K_m (the Michaelis constant). Along these lines, V_{max} is unchanged in competitive inhibition. As more substrate is added, the plots of a reaction taking place in the presence and absence of a competitive inhibitor advance towards the y-intercept until both plots converge on the same V_{max}. This is because the effects of a competitive inhibitor can be overcome at high substrate concentrations. Conversely, K_m is increased in competitive inhibition. This is because more substrate is needed for the reaction rate (V) to reach half its theoretical maximum value.

3.14. D (Hard)

K_m (the Michaelis constant) is unchanged and V_{max} (the theoretical maximum rate of reaction) is decreased in the Lineweaver-Burk plots of a reaction taking place in the presence and absence of a non-competitive inhibitor. V_{max} is decreased because in the presence of a non-competitive inhibitor, a proportion of enzymes will always be rendered inactive, due to conformational changes in the enzyme molecules. Contra to competitive inhibition this cannot be overcome by the addition of more substrate, as inhibitor and substrate molecules are not in direct competition with one another, since non-competitive inhibitors bind at a site distinct from the enzyme's active site. The Michaelis constant reflects the affinity of an enzyme's active site for its substrate. Along these lines, K_m is unchanged, as non-competitive inhibitors do not interfere with substrate binding to the enzyme's active site.

3.15. D (Moderate)

Raised serum enzyme levels can be indicative of a disease process associated with increased synthesis (including cellular proliferation). Likewise, increased serum enzyme activity can be attributed to the release of enzymes into the circulation due to cellular damage (cell death and cell membrane damage), as well as defective or unexpectedly slow clearance. In contrast, decreased enzyme activity or low serum enzyme levels can be linked to inborn errors of metabolism (IEM).

3.16. D (Moderate)

Elevated serum amylase is most likely to be seen in acute pancreatitis, as a result of injury to exocrine parenchyma and the concomitant leakage of this digestive enzyme. Acid phosphatase, an enzyme specifically found in the prostate, can be used as a diagnostic tool for prostatic carcinoma. Raised serum levels of the cardiac enzymes, creatine kinase (CK), glutamate-oxaloacetate transaminase (GOT) and lactate dehydrogenase (LDH) are indicative of an acute myocardial infarction (AMI). Likewise, hepatocyte damage leads to the release of alanine aminotransferase (ALT) and aspartate aminotransferase (AST). These are sensitive, but not specific as an index of liver injury. Although alanine aminotransferase is more specific for the liver than aspartate aminotransferase, as the latter is also found in muscle and erythrocytes (red blood cells).

3.17. A (Moderate)

Alpha-1-antitrypsin (AAT) is produced in the liver and excreted into serum where it serves to neutralise circulating proteolytic enzymes. Deficiency of this protease inhibitor thus makes individuals susceptible to emphysema, particularly if they are smokers. Alpha-1-antitrypsin is a major serum inhibiter of the neutrophil-derived, proteolytic enzyme elastase. Therefore, low serum levels of alpha-1-antitrypsin render lung tissue vulnerable to proteolysis by enzymes such as elastase, and have been linked to the pathogenesis of pulmonary emphysema.

3.18. B (Hard)

The first step in glycolysis involves the phosphorylation of glucose to glucose-6-phosphate. This reaction is catalysed by the enzyme hexokinase or glucokinase, and requires adenosine triphosphate (ATP). It also serves to fix glucose in the cell, as glucose cannot leave cells once in a phosphorylated form. In the second step of glycolysis, the enzyme phosphofructokinase (PFK) catalyses the conversion of fructose-6-phosphate to fructose-1,6-bisphosphate. This is the principal control step in glycolysis. The final step of glycolysis is catalysed by pyruvate kinase, and results in the formation of pyruvate from phosphoenolpyruvate (PEP). Glycogen phosphorylase catalyses the breakdown of glycogen (glycogenolysis), forming glucose-1-phosphate which is converted to glucose-6-phosphate and then enters the glycolytic pathway.

3.19. D (Easy)

Glycolysis is a nearly universal metabolic pathway which occurs in the cytosol of all cells. Adenosine triphosphate (ATP) is synthesised under aerobic and anaerobic conditions in this pathway. Accordingly, glycolysis is the only pathway capable of generating ATP in the absence of oxygen. Furthermore, glucagon inhibits this pathway by obstructing the enzymatic activity of phosphofructokinase (PFK) and pyruvate kinase.

3.20. B (Moderate)

The mitochondrial matrix enzyme pyruvate dehydrogenase (PDH) is controlled by phosphorylation. Along these lines, the dephosphorylated form of pyruvate dehydrogenase is active, and the phosphorylated form is inactive. The pyruvate dehydrogenase complex is also inhibited when energy levels are high. Accordingly, it is inactivated when there is a high cellular ratio of $NADH:NAD^+$.

3.21. A (Hard)

Citrate synthase, isocitrate dehydrogenase (IDH) and α-ketoglutarate dehydrogenase are key regulators of the Krebs cycle (tricarboxylic acid cycle). Citrate synthase is a key initiator enzyme which catalyses the irreversible condensation of oxaloacetate and acetyl-CoA to form citrate. Isocitrate dehydrogenase catalyses the oxidation of isocitrate to oxalosuccinate and subsequent decarboxylation of oxalosuccinate to α-ketoglutarate. Likewise, the oxidative decarboxylation of α-ketoglutarate to succinyl-CoA is catalysed by α-ketoglutarate dehydrogenase. In contrast, glycogen synthase is a key regulatory enzyme for glycogenesis.

3.22. C (Moderate)

The Krebs cycle (tricarboxylic acid cycle) takes place in the mitochondrial matrix. During each turn of the cycle, the reduced coenzymes NADH and $FADH_2$ are generated and carbon dioxide is released as a waste product. Furthermore, the cycle is inhibited by a high ATP: ADP ratio, and activated by a low ATP: ADP ratio.

3.23. D (Easy)

Cyanide inhibits complex IV (cytochrome c oxidase), the terminal component of the electron transport chain. This highly toxic agent prevents electrons from being released to oxygen as a terminal acceptor, and thus producing water. The signs and symptoms of cyanide poisoning are thus largely attributed to cellular hypoxia.

3.24. D (Hard)

Complexes I, III and IV pump protons (H^+) out of the mitochondrial matrix and across the inner mitochondrial membrane into the intermembrane space. Complex II, however, is not a proton pump as it does not traverse the inner mitochondrial membrane. Electrons enter the electron transport chain through complex I (donated by NADH) and complex II (donated by $FADH_2$). Moreover, as electrons move across the respiratory chain between complexes free energy is released.

CHAPTER 4
Clinical Genetics (MCQs)

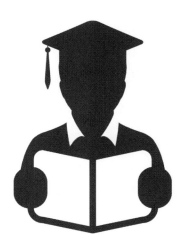

4.1. Which of the following terms is used to describe a pattern of inheritance in which the signs and symptoms of a genetic disorder become apparent at an earlier age in successive generations?

- A) Penetrance
- B) Expressivity
- C) Anticipation
- D) Lyonization

4.2. Which of the following conditions is **not** a triplet repeat disorder?

- A) Huntington's disease (HD)
- B) Myotonic dystrophy (MD)
- C) Fragile X syndrome (FXS)
- D) Alzheimer's disease (AD)

4.3. Tay-Sachs disease (TSD) is an autosomal recessive neurological disorder, most common in individuals of eastern European (Ashkenazi) Jewish descent. Katie's parents are both carriers for the disorder, what is the chance that Katie has Tay-Sachs disease?

- A) 25%
- B) 50%
- C) 75%
- D) 12.5%

4.4. Which of the following paradigms is typically seen in **dominantly** inherited diseases?

- A) Gain or alternation of function mutations
- B) Loss of function mutations
- C) Affected individuals may be compound heterozygous
- D) New mutations rates are low in comparison to recessive conditions

4.5. Which of the following genetic disorders is inherited in an autosomal **recessive** fashion?

A) Marfan syndrome (MS)
B) DiGeorge syndrome (22q11.2 deletion syndrome)
C) Myotonic dystrophy (MD)
D) Haemochromatosis

4.6. Which of the following genetic disorders is inherited in an autosomal **dominant** fashion?

A) Cystic Fibrosis (CF)
B) Achondroplasia
C) β-Thalassaemia
D) Sickle cell disease (SCD)

4.7. In X-linked inheritance:

A) Males tend to be affected more severely than females
B) Male to male transmission is not possible
C) Fragile X syndrome (FXS) is an example of X-linked dominant inheritance
D) All of the above

4.8. Haemophilia is an X-linked recessive condition. If an affected father and unaffected mother, who is not a carrier for the condition, give birth to a son what is the chance that he will have haemophilia?

A) 50%
B) 25%
C) 12.5%
D) 0%

4.9. The genetic code consists of 64 possible codons, of these 61 encode amino acids and 3 are stop codons. Which of the following triplets is **not** a stop codon?

A) UAG
B) UUA
C) UAA
D) UGA

4.10. Which of the following codons signals the **initiation** of protein synthesis?

A) AUG
B) AUU
C) AUA
D) AUC

4.11. Which of the following statements is **true** with regard to DNA structure and synthesis?

A) DNA is synthesised in a 5'-3' direction
B) DNA is synthesised in a 3'-5' direction
C) The sugar phosphate backbone in DNA consists of ribose sugars
D) Two parallel strands form a double helix in DNA

4.12. The structure of DNA is stabilised by hydrogen bonding between complementary purine and pyrimidine nucleotide bases. How many hydrogen bonds are formed between the bases guanine (G) and cytosine (C)?

A) Two
B) Three
C) Four
D) Five

4.13. In RNA, adenine (A) forms a base pair with:

A) Thymine (T)
B) Uracil (U)
C) Guanine (G)
D) Cytosine (C)

4.14. Mitochondrial DNA is inherited from:

A) Both parents
B) Mother only
C) Father only
D) Neither parent

4.15. Which of the following terms is used to describe mutations that alter the reading frame of DNA by the insertion or deletion of one or more bases?

A) Missense
B) Nonsense
C) Frameshift
D) Silent

4.16. The Hardy-Weinberg equation sets out the relationship between allele and genotype frequencies within a population at equilibrium. Which of the following statements is **true** with regard to the Hardy-Weinberg equation?

A) Allele frequencies can be estimated if genotype frequencies are known
B) Genotype frequencies can be estimated if allele frequencies are known
C) A and B
D) None of the above

4.17. The most common autosomal aneuploidies among humans include Patau syndrome, Edwards syndrome and Down's syndrome. Which of the following numerical chromosome abnormalities is seen in each of these syndromes?

A) Monosomy
B) Trisomy
C) Triploidy
D) Tetraploidy

4.18. Copy number variants (CNVs) are enriched in particular genomic regions. In which of the following genes would copy number variation (CNV) **not** be advantageous?

A) Immune response genes
B) Olfactory receptor genes
C) Transcriptional machinery and regulation genes
D) Sensory receptor genes

CHAPTER 4: Clinical Genetics (MCQs)

4.19. Karyotyping reveals the diploid complement of chromosomes in an individual. A normal **male** chromosome pattern would be described using which of the following karyotypes*?

*The number refers to the total number of chromosomes, while X and Y refer to sex chromosome constitution

A) 45, X
B) 47, XXY
C) 46, XX
D) 46, XY

4.20. Conventional cytogenetic analysis by G-banding (Giemsa banding) using light microscopy allows chromosomal aberrations to be detected during which stage of mitosis?

A) Prophase
B) Metaphase
C) Anaphase
D) Telophase

4.21. Cystic Fibrosis (CF) is caused by mutations in the following gene:

A) APC
B) BRCA1
C) BRCA2
D) CFTR

4.22. Hypercalcaemia is a clinical feature in which of the following disorders?

A) William's syndrome (WS)
B) DiGeorge syndrome (22q11.2 deletion syndrome)
C) Acute pancreatitis
D) Hypoparathyroidism

4.23. Which of the following is **not** a phase of the cell cycle?

- A) Mitosis
- B) Meiosis
- C) DNA Replication (S phase)
- D) Gap 2 (G_2)

4.24. Which of the following laboratory techniques for genetic testing is most likely to be used to identify a specific **known** mutation?

- A) Sanger sequencing
- B) Assays based on the polymerase chain reaction (PCR)
- C) Next generation (clonal) sequencing
- D) Karyotyping

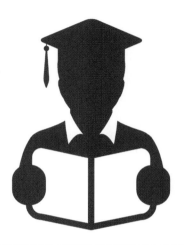

CHAPTER 4
Clinical Genetics (MCQs)

Answers and Detailed Solutions

The difficulty rating for each question (Easy, Moderate or Hard) can be found in parentheses next to the correct answer.

4.1. C (Moderate)

Genetic anticipation refers to a situation whereby the signs and symptoms of a genetic disorder become apparent at an earlier age in successive generations. Lyonization or X-inactivation involves the random and permanent inactivation of one of the X chromosomes in cells with more than one X chromosome. Expressivity indicates the degree to which a given phenotype is manifested by an individual. Likewise, penetrance refers to the frequency, usually expressed as a percentage, with which a particular genotype is expressed.

4.2. D (Hard)

Huntington's disease (HD), myotonic dystrophy (MD) and fragile X syndrome (FXS) are all triplet repeat disorders. These are caused by the expansion of trinucleotide repeats in certain genes (for example, Huntington's disease is caused by excessive CAG repeats in the HTT gene). In contrast, Alzheimer's disease (AD) is a heterogeneous polygenic disorder, for which numerous genetic and environmental influences have been identified.

4.3. A (Moderate)

In autosomal recessive disorders, the chance of two carriers having an affected child is 25%. This is contra to autosomal dominant diseases, in which the chance of passing on the mutation is 50%. Along these lines, homozygotes with two copies of the mutated gene will be affected in autosomal recessive inheritance, and heterozygotes with one copy of the mutated gene will be affected in autosomal dominant inheritance.

4.4. A (Hard)

Dominantly inherited diseases often result from gain or alteration of function mutations. In contrast, loss of function mutations are typically seen in recessive inheritance. New mutation rates are frequently higher for dominant disorders than recessive conditions. Moreover, affected individuals with recessively inherited diseases may be compound heterozygous (i.e. carry two different mutant alleles at a given locus).

4.5. D (Moderate)

The vast majority of cases of hereditary haemochromatosis or iron overload are inherited in an autosomal recessive fashion. Conversely, DiGeorge syndrome (22q11.2 deletion syndrome), myotonic dystrophy (MD) and Marfan syndrome (MS) are inherited in an autosomal dominant manner.

4.6. B (Moderate)

Achondroplasia is an autosomal dominant condition, often marked by rhizomelic (proximal) limb shortening. Cystic fibrosis (CF), Sickle cell disease (SCD) and β-Thalassaemia are inherited in an autosomal recessive fashion.

4.7. D (Moderate)

In X-linked inheritance, males tend to be affected more severely than females. Along these lines, only males are affected and females are carriers in X-linked recessive inheritance. This is contra to X-linked dominant inheritance, where males and females are both affected. It is important to note that male to male transmission is not possible regardless of whether it is X-linked dominant or recessive inheritance. In addition, fragile X syndrome (FXS) is an example of X-linked dominant inheritance.

4.8. D (Moderate)

In X-linked inheritance, male to male transmission is not possible. As such, there is 0% chance that the son will inherit haemophilia, as only his father is affected. If a man has an X-linked disorder all of his daughters will be carriers for the condition, while his sons will be unaffected (as there is no male to male transmission).

4.9. B (Easy)

There are three stop codons within the genetic code: UAA, UGA and UAG. Each of these codons functions as a signal for the termination of the translation process and thus the end of protein synthesis. The remaining 61 triplets encode the 20 naturally occurring amino acids.

4.10. A (Easy)

Protein synthesis (translation) begins with the start codon AUG, the triplet for Methionine (Met). The formation of an initiation complex involves the anticodon (UAC) of initiator transfer RNA (tRNA) binding, via complementary base pairing, to the start codon (AUG) on messenger RNA (mRNA). AUU, AUA and AUC encode the amino acid, Isoleucine (Ile).

4.11. A (Easy)

DNA or deoxyribonucleic acid is synthesised in a 5'-3' direction. The sugar phosphate backbone in DNA consists of deoxyribose sugars, while ribose is the sugar in the backbone of RNA. Likewise, two antiparallel strands form a double helix in DNA.

4.12. B (Easy)

The structure of DNA is stabilised by hydrogen bonding between complementary purine and pyrimidine nucleotide bases. In DNA, the purine bases include adenine (A) and guanine (G), and the pyrimidine bases include cytosine (C) and thymine (T). Three hydrogen bonds are formed between guanine and cytosine, and two hydrogen bonds are established between adenine and thymine. The presence of an additional hydrogen bond in the guanine-cytosine base pair makes it more stable than the adenine-thymine base pair.

4.13. B (Easy)

In DNA, thymine (T) pairs with adenine (A) whilst guanine (G) pairs with cytosine (C), via complementary Watson-Crick base pairing. In contrast, adenine (A) forms a base pair with uracil (U) in RNA.

4.14. B (Easy)

You inherit mitochondrial DNA from your mother only. Contra to sperm, ova contain lots of mitochondria. A clinical example of this maternal inheritance pattern is seen in maternally inherited diabetes and deafness (MIDD). This is a distinct subtype of diabetes, which is caused by a mutation in human mitochondrial DNA.

4.15. C (Moderate)

Frameshift mutations alter the reading frame of the DNA sequence by the insertion or deletion of one or more bases. This will often change the entire amino acid sequence from the position of the insertion or deletion, and may truncate the protein produced. Silent or neutral mutations do not alter the amino acid sequence. This phenomenon reflects the degeneracy of the genetic code, as the mutated and original codon encode the same amino acid. In nonsense mutations, a premature stop codon (UAA, UAG or UGA) is introduced, leading to the production of a truncated polypeptide. Missense mutations involve the substitution of one amino acid residue for another.

4.16. C (Hard)

The Hardy-Weinberg equation sets out the relationship between allele and genotype frequencies within a population at equilibrium. Along these lines, in an idealised population, allele frequencies can be estimated if genotype frequencies are known. Likewise, genotype frequencies can be estimated if allele frequencies are known.

4.17. B (Hard)

Patau syndrome, Edwards syndrome and Down's syndrome are all autosomal aneuploidies. The term aneuploidy describes a numerical chromosome abnormality in which there is the gain (trisomy) or loss (monosomy) of one or more chromosomes. The gain of a single chromosome is called trisomy, and is seen in Patau syndrome (Trisomy 13), Edwards syndrome (Trisomy 18) and Down's syndrome (Trisomy 21). Aneuploidies of every chromosome are possible, but individuals with these three are the least severely affected of the autosomal trisomies and are

CHAPTER 4: Clinical Genetics (MCQs)

thus capable of postnatal survival. These cytogenetic abnormalities do not affect the sex chromosomes (X and Y) as they are autosomal in nature, and an overlap is seen in the phenotype of each of these syndromes. Polyploidy refers to a numerical chromosome abnormality in which there is the gain of whole sets of chromosomes (triploidy or tetraploidy).

4.18. C (Hard)

Sensory receptor genes are enriched for copy number variants (CNVs). Olfactory receptor genes, for instance, have a very high rate of copy number variation (CNV). This variability is important as it allows us to distinguish between different smells. In like manner, copy number variation is advantageous in immune response genes, as it increases diversity and allows the immune system to respond to a wide-ranging number of pathogens. Conversely, transcriptional machinery and regulation genes tend to be copy number stable (CNS), as protein synthesis needs to be tightly regulated and controlled.

[Please bear in mind that the material covered in this question forms part of a burgeoning and ever-developing field of research, likely to offer considerable therapeutic benefit in years to come and, as such, represents the very limits of what would be expected of a pre-clinical medical student.]

4.19. D (Easy)

Klinefelter syndrome is associated with a 47, XXY karyotype, while individuals with Turner syndrome have a 45, X karyotype. Both of these chromosomal abnormalities are caused by anomalies in sex chromosome (X and Y) number. A normal female karyotype is designated as 46, XX and a normal male karyotype is written as 46, XY.

4.20. B (Hard)

The detection of chromosomal aberrations in conventional cytogenetic analysis by G-banding (Giemsa banding) is limited to metaphase chromosome spreads. In order to look at chromosome change, cells are allowed to divide and then arrested in the metaphase stage of the cell cycle by the addition of a mitotic spindle inhibitor. This is because DNA is highly coiled during metaphase, and thus visible down the microscope. Conversely, molecular cytogenetic analysis occurs at all stages of the cell cycle. Examples of molecular cytogenetic techniques include FISH (fluorescence in situ hybridisation), array CGH (microarray comparative genomic hybridisation) and MLPA (multiplex ligation-dependant probe amplification).

4.21. D (Easy)

Cystic Fibrosis (CF) is caused by mutations in the cystic fibrosis transmembrane conductance regulator (CFTR) gene. A germline mutation in the adenomatous polyposis coli (APC) tumour suppressor gene is implicated in familial adenomatous polyposis (FAP), an autosomal dominant cancer syndrome. In like manner, mutations in the tumour suppressor genes BRCA1 and BRCA2 are associated with breast and ovarian cancer.

4.22. A (Hard)

Hypercalcaemia is a clinical feature of William's syndrome (WS) or Williams-Beuren syndrome (WBS), due to disturbances in vitamin D metabolism. In contrast, hypocalcaemia is associated with DiGeorge syndrome (22q11.2 deletion syndrome), acute pancreatitis and hypoparathyroidism.

4.23. B (Moderate)

The five main phases of the cell cycle include: 2 gap phases (G_1 and G_2) and an S phase (DNA replication); these preparatory phases are collectively termed interphase, and are followed by the M (cell division) phase, which includes mitosis and cytokinesis. The 2 gap phases (G_1 and G_2) are checkpoints, which are important in maintaining the integrity of the replication process. During the first gap phase (G_1), numerous cellular components accumulate in preparation for DNA replication. This is followed by a synthesis (S) phase, in which there is a doubling up of the cell's total DNA content. The cell then undergoes further growth and metabolism (G_2) in preparation for mitosis (nuclear division) and cytokinesis (cytoplasmic division). Meiosis is a specialised reductive cell division, which leads to the formation of gametes (sperm and egg cells) and, as such, is not a phase of the cell cycle.

4.24. B (Hard)

If a specific mutation within a gene is **unknown**, gene sequencing, such as Sanger sequencing and next generation (clonal) sequencing, can be employed to identify the mutation. Additional discovery methods such as karyotyping can also be used if the identity of the mutation is unknown. In contrast, if the identity of the mutation is **known** then simple analytical methods can be deployed, such as assays based on the polymerase chain reaction (PCR).

CHAPTER 5
Embryology and Reproduction (MCQs)

5.1. Fertilisation age is used by clinicians to date pregnancy from the time at which fertilisation takes place. Under this system, pregnancy is divided into different periods of unequal length, which equate to major developmental events. Which of these periods is the longest?

A) Early development period
B) Embryonic (organogenesis) period
C) Foetal period
D) First trimester

5.2. The menstrual age is used by clinicians to date pregnancy from the woman's last menstrual period. Under this system, pregnancy is divided into three equal time periods (trimesters). How long does each trimester last?

A) 2 months
B) 3 months
C) 4 months
D) 5 months

5.3. The menstrual age is ___ week(s) more than the fertilisation age.

A) One
B) Two
C) Three
D) Four

5.4. Sperm must undergo which of the following processes as they migrate through the female reproductive tract **before** they can pass through the corona radiata and go on to reach the oocyte?

A) Fertilisation
B) Capacitation
C) The zona reaction
D) The acrosome reaction

5.5. After fertilisation, the zygote undergoes a series of rapid cell divisions collectively termed cleavage. Which of the following statements is **false** with regard to this embryological process?

A) Cleavage divisions are mitotic
B) The resulting daughter cells are called blastomeres or cleavage cells
C) It leads to the formation of a solid mass called a morula, which consists of 16-32 blastomeres
D) The zygote increases in size

5.6. During the second week of development, the inner cell mass (embryoblast) differentiates into a bilaminar embryonic disc composed of two cell layers: the epiblast and hypoblast. Which of the following statements is **true** with regard to this particular stage of embryonic development?

A) The epiblast forms the ventral surface of the embryo
B) The hypoblast forms the dorsal surface of the embryo
C) The amniotic cavity forms as a small fluid-filled cavity in the epiblast
D) All of the above

5.7. The developing syncytiotrophoblast of the placenta secretes human chorionic gonadotropin (hCG) not long after implantation has occurred. Which of the following statements is **true** with regard to this hormone?

A) It helps to maintain the endometrium
B) It is believed to contribute to maternal immunotolerance
C) It is used in pregnancy testing
D) All of the above

5.8. Which of the following processes is responsible for transformation of the bilaminar (two-layered) embryonic disc into a trilaminar (three-layered) disc consisting of three primary germ layers?

A) Gastrulation
B) Neurulation
C) Implantation
D) Placentation

5.9. Neurulation is the first event in the development of the central nervous system (CNS). Which of the following statements is **true** with regard to the process of neurulation and formation of the neural tube?

A) Neurulation is induced by signals originating from the notochord that cause the overlying mesoderm to thicken and form the neural plate
B) Fusion of the neural folds begins in the cervical region of the embryo
C) The caudal end of the neural tube will form the brain
D) All of the above

5.10. The process of neurulation is complete when the anterior and posterior neuropores fuse. Failure of the cranial end of the neural tube (the anterior neuropore) to fuse results in anencephaly. Which of the following statements is **false** with regard to this cranial neural tube defect (NTD)?

A) The forebrain is absent or severely hypoplastic
B) The brainstem is present
C) Reflex actions such as breathing are not possible
D) Anencephalic infants are often stillborn or die shortly after birth

5.11. Failure of the caudal end of the neural tube (the posterior neuropore) to fuse results in which of the following neural tube defects (NTDs)?

A) Rachischisis
B) Spina bifida (SB)
C) Encephalocele
D) Iniencephaly

5.12. During the fourth week of development, the embryo undergoes craniocaudal and lateral folding. Which of the following statements is **false** with regard to folding of the trilaminar embryonic disc in the craniocaudal and lateral axes?

A) Folding of the embryo is caused by the differential growth rate of various embryonic structures, such as the amniotic sac and the yolk sac
B) Ectopia cordis (EC) is caused by a failure in lateral folding
C) Gastroschisis is caused by a failure in craniocaudal folding
D) All of the above

5.13. The reproductive system is derived from the:

A) Endoderm
B) Intermediate mesoderm
C) Lateral plate mesoderm
D) Paraxial mesoderm

5.14. Which of the following statements is **true** with regard to the process of gametogenesis (spermatogenesis and oogenesis) and gonad development?

A) Male gametes (sperm) are produced by spermatogenesis from puberty onwards
B) All female gametes (oocytes) are present at birth
C) Male and female gonads are indistinguishable before the seventh week of embryonic development
D) All of the above

5.15. Which of the following terms is used to describe the failure of both or a single testis to descend from the abdominal cavity into the scrotum before birth?

A) Hydrocele
B) Epispadias
C) Hypospadias
D) Cryptorchidism

5.16. The diverse functions of the human placenta include:

A) Maternal-foetal exchange of oxygen and carbon dioxide
B) Selective acquisition of nutrients and the excretion of toxins
C) Production of the steroid hormones (oestrogen and progesterone)
D) All of the above

5.17. Which of the following statements is **false** with regard to luteinising hormone (LH):

A) High levels of estradiol (E_2) lead to a mid-cycle surge in the hormone that triggers ovulation, via positive feedback
3) It promotes development of the corpus luteum (CL), which secretes progesterone
C) It is produced by the posterior pituitary gland
D) All of the above

5.18. Which of the following statements is **false** with regard to follicle-stimulating hormone (FSH):

A) It stimulates follicular growth and maturation in the ovary
B) It stimulates granulosa cells to proliferate and produce estradiol (E_2)
C) It is produced by the anterior pituitary gland
D) Its production is stimulated by rising estradiol (E_2) levels, via negative feedback

5.19. The term teratogen is used to describe environmental factors that cause birth defects. Which of the following infectious, physical and chemical agents are teratogenic?

A) Cytomegalovirus (CMV)
B) Radiation
C) Pharmaceutical drugs
D) All of the above

5.20. Which of the following infectious agents commonly leads to the formation of skin lesions and scars in the newborn?

A) Herpes simplex virus (HSV)
B) *Escherichia coli (E. coli)*
C) Human immunodeficiency virus (HIV)
D) Hepatitis B virus (HBV)

5.21. If Rubella (German measles) is contracted by a mother during the early stages of pregnancy it can cause which of the following birth defects?

A) Cataracts and hearing loss
B) Microcephaly and cardiac defects
C) A and B
D) None of the above

5.22. Maternal infection with toxoplasmosis during the first trimester of pregnancy can cause a number birth defects. The causative agent in toxoplasmosis is a:

A) Parasite
B) Bacterium
C) Virus
D) Fungus

5.23. Which of the following neonatal infections is typically acquired during passage through the birth canal?

A) Gonorrhoea
B) Cytomegalovirus (CMV)
C) Toxoplasmosis
D) Varicella-zoster virus (VZV)

5.24. Which of the following statements is **false** with regard to the drug thalidomide?

A) Originally used as a drug for morning sickness
B) Causes limb malformations
C) Currently used to alleviate the symptoms of human immunodeficiency virus (HIV) and leprosy in certain countries
D) Can be protective against birth defects

CHAPTER 5

Embryology and Reproduction (MCQs)

Answers and Detailed Solutions

The difficulty rating for each question (Easy, Moderate or Hard) can be found in parentheses next to the correct answer.

5.1. C (Hard)

The first two weeks after fertilisation are known as the early development or pre-embryonic period. This period of cell division is followed by the embryonic or organogenesis period (weeks 3-8). It is during this time that most of the embryo's internal organs are formed. The longest period is the foetal period, this lasts from week 9 up until birth. This involves the growth and maturation of the organs formed during organogenesis.

5.2. B (Easy)

Clinicians divide human gestation into three equal trimesters, which each last 3 months. The average human gestational period is approximately 40 weeks from the woman's last menstrual period (menstrual age).

5.3. B (Easy)

Two weeks elapse between the woman's last menstrual period (menstrual age) and fertilisation (fertilisation age). This is because fertilisation cannot occur until mid-cycle (around day 14 in a 28-day menstrual cycle), as this is when ovulation occurs and an oocyte is released. The menstrual age is thus two weeks more than the fertilisation age. The average human gestational period is approximately 38 weeks from fertilisation (fertilisation age).

5.4. B (Moderate)

As sperm migrate through the female reproductive tract, they are modified and mature in a process known as capacitation. Once capacitated sperm can pass through the corona radiata and go on to reach the oocyte. The head of the sperm cell has a special region called the acrosome. This contains hydrolytic enzymes which are released in order to break down the zona pellucida in the acrosome reaction. Capacitation and the acrosome reaction are essential for fertilisation (the fusion of male and female gametes). The nucleus of the sperm can then enter the oocyte. Following this, the zona pellucida will secrete an enzyme to prevent further sperm from entering the oocyte. This process is known as the zona reaction, and it ensures that only one sperm nucleus enters the oocyte.

5.5. D (Moderate)

The zygote does not increase in size during cleavage, rather the cells (blastomeres) get progressively smaller after each cell division. These cleavage divisions are mitotic, and produce identical daughter cells called blastomeres or cleavage cells. This series of rapid cells divisions eventually leads to the formation of a solid mass called a morula, which consists of 16-32 blastomeres.

5.6. C (Hard)

During the second week of development, the inner cell mass (embryoblast) divides into two cell layers (the epiblast and hypoblast), and the dorsal/ventral axis of the embryo is established. This is the first stage of organisation in terms of the body plan in embryonic development. The epiblast forms the **dorsal** surface of the embryo, while the hypoblast forms the **ventral** surface of the embryo. The amniotic cavity then forms as a small fluid-filled cavity in the epiblast, and the hypoblast forms the yolk sac. The bilaminar embryonic disc thus lies between the amniotic cavity and the yolk sac.

5.7. D (Moderate)

During the second week of development, the outer cell mass (trophoblast) differentiates into two tissues: the outer syncytiotrophoblast and inner cytotrophoblast. The developing syncytiotrophoblast of the placenta secretes human chorionic gonadotropin (hCG) not long after implantation has occurred. This helps to maintain the endometrium so that it is not shed as part of the menstrual cycle, and thus assists in sustaining early pregnancy. The hormone is also used in pregnancy testing, as its presence or absence can be detected in maternal urine or serum. In addition, it is believed to contribute to maternal immunotolerance towards the implanted embryo.

CHAPTER 5: Embryology and Reproduction (MCQs)

5.8. A (Hard)

Gastrulation commences in week three with the appearance of the primitive steak and is responsible for transformation of the bilaminar (two-layered) embryonic disc into a trilaminar (three-layered) disc. At the end of gastrulation we are left with a trilaminar structure composed of three primary germ layers: ectoderm, mesoderm and endoderm, each derived from the epiblast cells of the bilaminar embryo.

5.9. B (Hard)

Neurulation is induced by signals originating from the notochord that cause the overlying ectoderm (not mesoderm) to thicken and form the neural plate, which is flat. The lateral edges of the neural plate then lift up to form neural folds, which will go on to fuse in the midline and form the neural tube. Fusion of the neural folds begins in the cervical region of the embryo. Once this process is complete, the caudal end of the neural tube will form the spinal cord and the cranial end of the neural tube will form the brain.

5.10. C (Hard)

Failure of the cranial end of the neural tube (the anterior neuropore) to fuse results in anencephaly (without a brain). No forebrain structures develop, or the forebrain is severely hypoplastic. In contrast, the caudal end of the neural tube does form, so the brainstem is often present and functional. The primitive, life-supporting functions of the brain (such as respiration and heart rate) reside in the brain stem. Accordingly, it is possible for infants with anencephaly to sustain reflex actions such as breathing, albeit normally only for a short period of time. Anencephaly is a devastating congenital malformation and, as such, affected infants are often stillborn or die shortly after birth.

5.11. A (Hard)

Failure of the caudal end of the neural tube (the posterior neuropore) to fuse results in rachischisis (or cleft vertebral column). In this congenital anomaly, neural tissue is left exposed to the external environment (resulting in a high risk of infection), and the spinal cord fails to form properly leading to paralysis. Rachischisis is commonly described as the most severe form of spina bifida (SB). In essence, rachischisis is a failure of the neural tube to form, while spina bifida is a failure of the vertebrae to form correctly. Spina bifida is caused by abnormal induction of the sclerotome by the notochord. There are various degrees of severity, these include: spina bifida occulta (SBO), meningocele and myelomeningocele. Encephalocele is a neural tube defect (NTD) indicated by herniation of the intracranial contents through a bony defect in the cranium. Iniencephaly is a rare and lethal neural tube defect characterised by congenital absence of the neck (inion) and severe retroflexion of the head.

5.12. C (Hard)

During the fourth week of development, embryonic folding occurs due to the differential growth rate of various embryonic structures, including the amniotic sac and the yolk sac. The amniotic sac, for instance, undergoes rapid enlargement while the yolk sac remains a similar size. Ectopia cordis (EC) and gastroschisis are both ventral body wall defects, caused by a failure in lateral folding. In ectopia cordis, the lateral folds fail to fuse in the thoracic region, leaving the heart on the outside of the body and exposed to the external environment and thus at high risk of infection. Similarly, in gastroschisis the lateral folds fail to fuse in the abdominal region, leaving the abdominal organs (such as the intestines) on the outside of the body.

5.13. B (Hard)

The mesoderm becomes highly organised in the early stages of embryonic development, and differentiates into three parts: paraxial mesoderm (either side of the midline), intermediate mesoderm (in the middle), and the lateral plate mesoderm (on the lateral edge). The reproductive system is derived from the intermediate mesoderm, while the dermis of skin and most of the skeleton and the skeletal muscles that attach to the skeleton are derived from paraxial mesoderm. Likewise, the lining of body cavities (such as the abdominal and thoracic cavities) are derived from the lateral plate mesoderm.

CHAPTER 5: Embryology and Reproduction (MCQs)

5.14. D (Easy)

Male and female gonads become distinguishable at the end of the seventh week of embryonic development, as they differentiate based on the presence or absence of a Y chromosome. With regard to gametogenesis, male gametes (sperm) are produced by spermatogenesis after puberty, while all female gametes (oocytes) are present at birth.

5.15. D (Moderate)

Cryptorchidism describes the failure of both or a single testis to descend from the abdominal cavity into the scrotum before birth. Epispadias and Hypospadias are both due to abnormal development of the external genitalia. Epispadias is a rare congenital abnormality that occurs when the urethra opens on the upper side (dorsal surface) of the penis, and is often associated with exstrophy of the bladder. Hypospadias is a congenital anomaly in which the urethra opens on the ventral surface of the penis, due to incomplete fusion of the urethral folds during development. A hydrocele is a fluid filled cyst caused by a patent processus vaginalis (PPV). It is formed by clear fluid and, as such, light can pass through it easily.

5.16. D (Easy)

The human placenta is responsible for a number of diverse functions. These include, but are not limited to, maternal-foetal exchange of oxygen and carbon dioxide, the selective acquisition of nutrients and the excretion of toxins, and the production of steroid hormones (oestrogen and progesterone).

5.17. C (Moderate)

Luteinising hormone (LH) is produced by the anterior (not the posterior) pituitary gland. High levels of estradiol (E_2) lead to a mid-cycle surge in the hormone that triggers ovulation once the oocyte is ready, via positive feedback. Moreover, luteinising hormone promotes development of the corpus luteum (CL), which secretes progesterone.

5.18. D (Moderate)

The production of follicle-stimulating hormone (FSH), along with gonadotropin-releasing hormone (GnRH) and luteinising hormone (LH), is inhibited (not stimulated) by rising estradiol (E_2) levels, via negative feedback. Follicle-stimulating hormone is also responsible for stimulating follicular growth and maturation in the ovary, and the promotion of estradiol (E_2) production from granulosa cells. Furthermore, the hormone is produced by the anterior pituitary gland.

5.19. D (Easy)

Infectious agents such as cytomegalovirus (CMV), physical agents such as radiation and chemical agents such as pharmaceutical drugs would all be classified as teratogens, as each of these environmental factors has the potential to disrupt embryonic development and cause birth defects. If a mother is infected with cytomegalovirus during pregnancy, for instance, the virus can pass to the foetus and potentially cause microcephaly (an abnormally small brain), microphthalmia (underdeveloped or small eyes), cerebral calcification, and intrauterine growth retardation (the baby is very small at birth).

5.20. A (Easy)

Infants born to women with herpes simplex virus (HSV) may develop skin lesions and scars, as the virus is transmitted to the newborn in the mother's infected birth canal during delivery.

5.21. C (Easy)

Rubella (German measles) is a highly contagious childhood virus. If it is contracted by a mother during the early stages of pregnancy it can cause a number of birth defects. These include, but are not limited to, microcephaly (an abnormally small brain), cardiac defects, cataracts and hearing loss (as the virus affects formation of the infant's ears).

5.22. A (Moderate)

The causative agent in toxoplasmosis, *Toxoplasma gondii (T. gondii)*, is an obligate intracellular protozoan parasite. Infection with this protozoan disease during the first trimester of pregnancy can cause a number of birth defects. These include, but are not limited to, microcephaly (an abnormally small brain), hydrocephaly (water on the brain) and microphthalmia (underdeveloped or small eyes). This is contra to the vast majority of infectious agents that cause birth defects, as these are often viral in nature.

5.23. A (Moderate)

Cytomegalovirus (CMV), toxoplasmosis and varicella-zoster virus (the causative agent of chickenpox and shingles) are typically transmitted to the foetus during pregnancy (in utero). In contrast, *Neisseria gonorrhoeae (N. gonorrhoeae)* is typically acquired by infants during passage through the birth canal.

5.24. D (Easy)

Thalidomide is a pharmaceutical agent widely used in the middle of the twentieth century as a treatment for morning sickness. Its use was discontinued after it was found that the drug caused birth defects, particularly affecting the upper and lower limbs. It is currently used, however, in countries such as Brazil to help manage the symptoms of leprosy and human immunodeficiency virus (HIV).

CHAPTER 6
The Respiratory System (MCQs)

6.1. The respiratory tract can be functionally divided into conducting and respiratory portions. Which of these structures is found in **both** the conducting and respiratory portions of the respiratory tract?

- A) Trachea
- B) Respiratory Bronchioles
- C) Nasopharynx
- D) Nasal Cavity

6.2. The respiratory tract can be anatomically divided into upper and lower compartments. Which of these structures is found in the **upper** respiratory tract?

- A) Alveoli
- B) Trachea
- C) Larynx
- D) Main (primary) bronchi

6.3. The left and right lungs are divided into lobes, which are separated from one another by interlobar fissures. How many lobes are there in the **right** lung?

- A) Two
- B) Three
- C) Four
- D) Five

6.4. Rank the different components of the tracheobronchial tree in order of size, from smallest to largest:

- A) Terminal bronchioles, bronchioles, respiratory bronchioles, lobar (secondary) bronchi, segmental (tertiary) bronchi, main (primary) bronchi, trachea
- B) Respiratory bronchioles, terminal bronchioles, bronchioles, segmental (tertiary) bronchi, lobar (secondary) bronchi, main (primary) bronchi, trachea
- C) Respiratory bronchioles, terminal bronchioles, lobar (secondary) bronchi, segmental (tertiary) bronchi, main (primary) bronchi, bronchioles, trachea
- D) Respiratory bronchioles, terminal bronchioles, bronchioles, main (primary) bronchi, lobar (secondary) bronchi, segmental (tertiary) bronchi, trachea

6.5. A number of important structures pass through the diaphragm at various thoracic vertebral levels (T1-T12). Which of the following statements is **false** with regard to the level at which these structures penetrate the diaphragm?

A) The descending thoracic aorta passes through at T12 to become the abdominal aorta
B) The thoracic duct passes through at T10
C) The oesophagus and vagus nerves pass through at T10
D) The inferior vena cava (IVC) and right phrenic nerve pass through at T8

6.6. Airflow during inspiration and expiration depends on the pressure gradient set up between atmospheric (barometric) pressure (P_B) and alveolar pressure (P_A). Air will be drawn into the lungs when:

A) $P_B > P_A$
B) $P_A > P_B$
C) $P_B < P_A$
D) $P_B = P_A$

6.7. Which of the following statements is **false** with regard to the action of the ventilatory muscles during **inspiration**?

A) External intercostal muscles contract
B) Internal intercostal muscles contract
C) Diaphragm muscles contract
D) Neck muscles contract

6.8. Which of the following statements is **false** with regard to the action of the ventilatory muscles during **expiration**?

A) External intercostal muscles relax
B) Internal intercostal muscles contract
C) Diaphragm muscles relax
D) Abdominal wall muscles relax

6.9. The pattern of airflow through the respiratory system affects the work of breathing. Airflow can be laminar, turbulent or a mixture of the two (transitional flow). Which of the following statements is **false** with regard to the types of airflow that occur in the lung?

  A) Laminar flow is organised with a parabolic velocity profile, while turbulent flow is disorganised with a flat velocity profile
  B) Turbulent flow is more energy-efficient than laminar flow
  C) A low Reynolds number (Re) indicates laminar flow
  D) A high Reynolds number (Re) indicates turbulent flow

6.10. Which of the following respiratory disorders is an example of a **restrictive** pulmonary disease?

  A) Asthma
  B) Pulmonary fibrosis
  C) Chronic obstructive pulmonary disease (COPD)
  D) None of the above

6.11. Which of the following diseases is associated with **increased** lung compliance?

  A) Emphysema
  B) Kyphoscoliosis
  C) Third-degree circumferential burns
  D) Pulmonary fibrosis

6.12. Pulmonary surfactant is secreted by:

  A) Goblet cells
  B) Type I pneumocytes
  C) Type II pneumocytes
  D) Alveolar Macrophages

6.13. Hyperventilation can lead to which of the following acid-base abnormalities?

  A) Respiratory Acidosis
  B) Respiratory Alkalosis
  C) Metabolic Acidosis
  D) Metabolic Alkalosis

6.14. Chronic obstructive pulmonary disease (COPD) can lead to which of the following acid-base abnormalities?

A) Respiratory Acidosis
B) Respiratory Alkalosis
C) Metabolic Acidosis
D) Metabolic Alkalosis

6.15. Which of the following is **not** a compensatory physiological change seen at high altitude?

A) Polycythaemia
B) Hyperventilation
C) Decreased 2,3-diphosphoglycerate (2,3-DPG)
D) Increased 2,3-diphosphoglycerate (2,3-DPG)

6.16. An umbrella term for emphysema and chronic bronchitis:

A) Bronchiectasis
B) Chronic obstructive pulmonary disease (COPD)
C) Sarcoidosis
D) Primary ciliary dyskinesia (PCD) or Kartagener's Syndrome (KS)

6.17. The approach to clinical treatment is the **same** for the following two respiratory disorders:

A) Asthma and chronic obstructive pulmonary disease (COPD)
B) Chronic obstructive pulmonary disease (COPD) and pulmonary fibrosis
C) Emphysema and sarcoidosis
D) Interstitial lung disease and asthma

6.18. Which of the following terms is used to describe the volume of gas moved in or out of the lungs during quiet (normal) breathing?

A) Tidal volume (TV)
B) Inspiratory reserve volume (IRV)
C) Expiratory reserve volume (ERV)
D) Residual volume (RV)

CHAPTER 6: The Respiratory System (MCQs)

6.19. Lung capacities are the combination or sum of two or more of the four standard lung volumes (tidal volume, inspiratory reserve volume, expiratory reserve volume and residual volume). Functional residual capacity (FRC) describes the volume of gas contained in the lungs after a normal expiration. This capacity would be calculated from which of the following combinations?

  A) TV + IRV + ERV
  B) TV + IRV + ERV + RV
  C) ERV + RV
  D) TV + IRV

6.20. Peak expiratory flow rate (PEFR) is a convenient index of airway obstruction. Which of the following statements is **false** with regard to this objective measure of respiratory obstruction?

  A) Peak flow meters are routinely used in clinical practice to measure PEFR
  B) Diurnal variation is common in PEFR readings
  C) It can be used to help diagnose and monitor asthma
  D) It can be used to help diagnose and monitor pulmonary fibrosis

6.21. The maturation of the lungs is divided into four histologic developmental stages: pseudoglandular, canalicular, terminal sac and alveolar. The **earliest** phase at which foetal survival is possible is the:

  A) Pseudoglandular period
  B) Canalicular period
  C) Terminal sac period
  D) Alveolar period

6.22. The size, density and shape of inhaled particles determines their site of deposition in the respiratory tract. Particle deposition occurs via a number of different mechanisms, including inertial impaction, sedimentation and diffusion. Which of the following particles would be deposited in the bronchioles by the mechanism of **sedimentation**?

  A) Pollen
  B) Sawdust
  C) Fungal spores
  D) Asbestos

6.23. Which of the following clinical symptoms is **not** associated with lung cancer?

A) Dyspnoea
B) Haemoptysis
C) Weight gain
D) Chest pain

6.24. A number of different pathological fluids can accumulate in the pleural cavity (the potential space between the visceral and parietal pleura). Which of the following terms is used to describe the presence of excess fluid in the pleural cavity?

A) Pleural effusion
B) Haemothorax
C) Empyema
D) Pneumothorax

CHAPTER 6

The Respiratory System (MCQs)

Answers and Detailed Solutions

The difficulty rating for each question (Easy, Moderate or Hard) can be found in parentheses next to the correct answer.

6.1. B (Moderate)

Respiratory bronchioles are transition structures that straddle the conducting and respiratory portions of the respiratory tract and, as such, they both conduct air and participate in gaseous exchange. In contrast, the trachea, nasal cavity and nasopharynx are all part of the conducting portion of the respiratory tract, and thus involved in delivering air to the respiratory portion of the respiratory tract for the purpose of gaseous exchange.

6.2. C (Easy)

The larynx is found in the upper respiratory tract, while the trachea, main (primary) bronchi and alveoli are all found in the lower respiratory tract. The anatomical division of the respiratory tract into upper and lower compartments can also be used clinically to classify respiratory tract infections (RTIs). Pneumonia, for instance, is classed as a lower respiratory tract infection (LRTI), while the common cold is classified as an upper respiratory tract infection (URTI).

6.3. B (Easy)

There are three lobes in the right lung, separated by an oblique and horizontal fissure, and two lobes in the left lung, separated by an oblique fissure. These lobes are further subdivided into numerous segments (for example, the lower lobe of the right lung contains a superior, anterior basal, lateral basal and posterior basal segment).

6.4. B (Moderate)

The trachea bifurcates into the left and right main (primary) bronchi at the carina. Primary bronchi then branch into the appropriate lobes of the lung, forming lobar (secondary) bronchi, which in turn divide into segmental (tertiary) bronchi. Branching then continues to form the bronchioles, terminal bronchioles and finally the respiratory bronchioles. For further information about the respiratory bronchioles refer to the detailed solution for question 6.1. in this chapter.

6.5. B (Moderate)

The descending thoracic aorta passes through the diaphragm at vertebral level T12 to become the abdominal aorta. Likewise, the thoracic duct passes through the diaphragm at vertebral level T12 (not T10), while the oesophagus and vagus nerves pass through the diaphragm at vertebral level T10. The inferior vena cava (IVC) and right phrenic nerve pass through the diaphragm at vertebral level T8.

6.6. A (Moderate)

In order to generate movement of air into the lungs, we need to create a negative intrathoracic pressure (ITP). Therefore, during the process of inspiration the barometric pressure is greater than the alveolar pressure ($P_B > P_A$). Similarly, in order to generate movement of air out of the lungs, we need to create a positive intrathoracic pressure. As such, during the process of expiration the alveolar pressure is greater than the barometric pressure ($P_A > P_B$).

6.7. B (Easy)

Inspiration in normal (quiet) breathing is primarily diaphragmatic. The diaphragm muscles contract and the diaphragm flattens. In addition, the external intercostal muscles help to stabilise the rib cage. With increasing effort, for instance when exercising, the external intercostal muscles contract, which leads to the expansion and elevation of the rib cage. Moreover, during laboured breathing the neck muscles contract and the accessory muscles and shoulder girdle muscles are brought into action to aid inspiration. Conversely, the internal intercostal muscles will be relaxed during inspiration.

CHAPTER 6: The Respiratory System (MCQs)

6.8. D (Easy)

Expiration in normal (quiet) breathing is largely due to the elastic recoil of lung tissue and structures of the thoracic wall. Accordingly, the diaphragm muscles relax and return to their normal position. Likewise, the external intercostal muscles relax during expiration. With increasing effort, the internal intercostal muscles contract pulling the ribs inwards and downwards to their original position. Similarly, the abdominal wall muscles contract, which pushes the abdominal contents up against the diaphragm and helps to push the diaphragm upwards into the thoracic cavity.

6.9. B (Hard)

Reynolds number (Re) indicates whether flow is turbulent or laminar. A low Reynolds number denotes laminar flow (Re < 2000), while a high Reynolds number demonstrates turbulent flow (Re > 2000). Laminar flow is organised with a parabolic velocity profile, while turbulent flow is disorganised with a flat velocity profile and, as such, laminar flow is more energy-efficient than turbulent flow.

6.10. B (Easy)

Pulmonary fibrosis is a restrictive pulmonary disease, as the lung volume available for gaseous exchange is reduced. Conversely, in obstructive pulmonary diseases, like asthma and chronic obstructive pulmonary disease (COPD), the lung volume available for gaseous exchange remains unchanged, while the flow of gases along the airways is obstructed.

6.11. A (Hard)

Kyphoscoliosis, third-degree circumferential burns and pulmonary fibrosis are all associated with decreased compliance of the lung. In patients with third-degree circumferential burns, the skin becomes very tight and loses its elastic qualities. This burnt tissue (eschar) thus acts like a rubber band around the chest making breathing extremely difficult. Similarly, in chest wall deformities such as kyphoscoliosis, breathing can be challenging due to reduced lung compliance. In pleural or interstitial pulmonary fibrosis, compliance is also reduced, as the elastic tissue of the lungs is replaced by fibrotic tissue. Conversely, in emphysema lung compliance is increased, albeit at the expense of alveolar exchange. Emphysema is marked by widespread destruction and dilatation of the distal airways. As such, while it is very easy to breath, destruction of the alveolar-capillary interface leads to very little gaseous exchange and hypoxia.

6.12. C (Moderate)

Type II pneumocytes secrete pulmonary surfactant, which acts a detergent and lowers alveolar surface tension. This helps to improve pulmonary compliance, and ensures that alveoli remain open during respiration (i.e. prevents atelectasis). A deficiency in the production of pulmonary surfactant results in respiratory distress syndrome (RDS). Type I pneumocytes are squamous epithelial cells, and are responsible for gaseous exchange. Alveolar macrophages are part of the innate immune system, and ingest any foreign material (e.g. dust or carbon) that is deposited in the lungs, in order to help maintain the sterility of the lung environment. The primary role of goblet cells is to secrete mucus. The viscosity of mucus is thus largely dependant on contributions from goblet cells, as well as seromucous glands.

6.13. B (Hard)

Hyperventilation is one of the most common causes of respiratory alkalosis (pH > 7.45). Respiratory alkalosis results from hyperventilation, as increased carbon dioxide excretion leads to hypocapnia (a low carbon dioxide level). Hyperventilation can be due to anxiety (e.g. a panic attack), a physiological response seen at high altitude, iatrogenic (caused by medical professionals or procedures), or a normal stress response.

6.14. A (Hard)

Chronic obstructive pulmonary disease (COPD) is a common cause of respiratory acidosis (pH < 7.35). Respiratory acidosis is seen in conditions, such as COPD, where carbon dioxide is retained due to inadequate ventilation. Carbon dioxide can also accumulate due to parenchymal lung disease and inadequate perfusion. In addition, respiratory acidosis is a common side-effect of morphine use, as this analgesic agent can cause opioid-induced respiratory depression. If this occurs, the opioid antagonist naloxone can be administered to reverse morphine's respiratory depressant action.

6.15. C (Hard)

Acclimatisation at high altitude is marked by a number of compensatory physiological changes. There is a rightward shift of the Hb-O_2 dissociation curve, which causes haemoglobin to offload oxygen more readily into tissues. This is mediated by an increase in 2,3-diphosphoglycerate (2,3-DPG), which causes enhanced unloading of oxygen. In order to remove carbon dioxide from the circulation and make space for oxygen, hyperventilation also occurs, which results in hypocapnia (low carbon dioxide levels) and leads to respiratory alkalosis. In addition, there is an increase in the number of red blood cells (polycythaemia), in order to assist with oxygen transport. This leads to an increase in blood viscosity, however, which can precipitate thrombotic complications.

6.16. B (Easy)

Chronic obstructive pulmonary disease (COPD) is an umbrella term for chronic bronchitis and emphysema. Chronic bronchitis is marked by mucus gland hyperplasia, manifested clinically as mucus hypersecretion, secondary bacterial infection by low virulence organisms and chronic inflammation. Emphysema is characterised by alveolar wall weakness and destruction, caused by chronic inflammation of the small airways of the lung. Moreover, bronchiectasis is clinically distinguished by irreversible enlargement of the bronchi and bronchioles due to destruction of the muscles and elastic tissue, and is often precipitated by infection. Sarcoidosis is an idiopathic multi-system disease of young women, associated with the formation of non-caseating pulmonary granulomas that can lead to fibrosis. In addition, Kartagener's syndrome (KS) or primary ciliary dyskinesia (PCD) is an autosomal recessive genetic disorder made apparent by abnormalities in respiratory cilia and sperm flagella, and concomitant issues with mucociliary function and fertility.

6.17. A (Moderate)

Clinicians adopt a similar approach to the treatment of asthma and chronic obstructive pulmonary disease (COPD), as they are both obstructive pulmonary diseases and accordingly characterised by airflow limitation. Bronchodilator therapy, for instance, is routinely used in the clinical management of asthma and COPD. Sympathomimetic agents such as selective β_2 agonists, both short acting (e.g. albuterol-salbutamol) and long acting (e.g. salmeterol), can thus be administered to patients with these respiratory disorders. Likewise, corticosteroid therapy can serve as a non-specific pharmacological treatment for asthma and COPD, as it helps to dampen down the immune response in the airways. Although the approach to clinical treatment is the same for these two respiratory disorders, it is important to note that while airflow limitation is reversible in asthma, it is irreversible in COPD.

6.18. A (Moderate)

There are four standard lung volumes (tidal volume, inspiratory reserve volume, expiratory reserve volume and residual volume), which can be measured using a spirometer. Tidal volume (TV) is used to describe the volume of gas moved in or out of the lungs during quiet (normal) breathing. Inspiratory reserve volume (IRV) refers to the maximal volume of air that can be forcefully inhaled over and above the tidal volume. Expiratory reserve volume (ERV) refers to the maximal volume of air that can be forcefully exhaled over and above the tidal volume. Residual volume (RV) is the air that remains in the lungs after a maximal expiration. This is the only lung volume that cannot be measured by spirometry.

6.19. C (Hard)

Functional residual capacity (FRC) describes the volume of gas contained in the lungs after a normal expiration, and is determined from the following combination: ERV + RV. Total lung capacity (TLC) is calculated from the sum of all four lung volumes: TV + IRV + ERV + RV. Vital capacity (VC) is calculated from the following combination: TV + IRV + ERV. In like manner, inspiratory capacity (IC) refers to the sum of TV and IRV.

6.20. D (Easy)

Peak expiratory flow rate (PEFR) provides a convenient measure of airway obstruction. PEFR can be used by clinicians to help diagnose and monitor asthma, as it is an obstructive pulmonary disease and thus characterised by airflow limitation. In contrast, PEFR is not used to help with the diagnosis and management of pulmonary fibrosis as this is a restrictive pulmonary disease, and PEFR is specifically used to measure airflow obstruction. Diurnal variation is common in PEFR readings, with the lowest readings in the morning and the highest readings in the evening. Moreover, peak flow meters are routinely used in everyday clinical practice to measure PEFR.

6.21. B (Hard)

The maturation and development of the lungs is a highly significant determinant of prognosis at birth. The histologic developmental stage reached by the infant (pseudoglandular, canalicular, terminal sac or alveolar) is thus particularly important for premature births. The pseudoglandular period (5-17 weeks) involves the branching of the respiratory tree to form terminal bronchioles. At this point in development only the conducting portion of the respiratory tract has been formed. Respiration is therefore not possible, as the respiratory portion of the respiratory tract is absent, and a foetus will not survive if born at this stage. The earliest phase at which foetal survival is possible is the canalicular period (16-25 weeks). This phase of lung maturation involves the first appearance of the respiratory portion of the respiratory tract and, as such, is the first point in development at which gaseous exchange can potentially take place. During this period, the terminal bronchioles give rise to respiratory bronchioles, which then go on to form alveolar ducts. Respiration is possible at this developmental stage, although the lungs are still very immature so there is a low chance of foetal survival. The further the infant is towards the end of the canicular period (i.e. 24-25 weeks), the better the chances of foetal survival. During the terminal sac period (26 weeks to birth), further terminal sacs (primitive alveoli) develop and the capillaries are brought into close proximity with the respiratory epithelium, forming a blood-air barrier. The respiratory epithelium contains cells which differentiate to give rise to type I and II pneumocytes, which act as an interface for gaseous exchange and secrete pulmonary surfactant respectively. The amount of pulmonary surfactant produced is an important determinant of foetal survival during this period, as if surfactant is not produced in sufficient quantities the infant's alveoli will start to collapse. The alveolar period (36 weeks to middle childhood) is the final stage of lung maturation, and primarily occurs postnatally. This is because the vast majority of mature alveoli develop after birth, and keep on growing until middle childhood (around 8 years of age).

6.22. D (Hard)

Very Large particles (>8μm) such as pollen and sawdust, are deposited in the nose and pharynx by the mechanism of inertial impaction. Likewise, large particles (3-8 μm) such as fungal spores, are deposited in the large airways by the mechanism of inertial impaction. In contrast, small particles (0.5-3 μm) such as asbestos and particulate matter (pm), are deposited in the bronchioles by the mechanism of sedimentation.

6.23. C (Easy)

Dyspnoea (shortness of breath), haemoptysis (coughing up blood) and chest pain are all clinical symptoms associated with lung cancer. Conversely, individuals with lung cancer often experience weight loss, as opposed to weight gain, as a nonspecific symptom of malignancy.

6.24. A (Moderate)

A pleural effusion refers to the presence of excess fluid in the pleural cavity (the potential space between the visceral and parietal pleura). Haemothorax describes the accumulation of blood in the pleural cavity, usually due to trauma or a ruptured thoracic aortic aneurysm. Similarly, the presence of pus in the pleural cavity is known as an empyema or pyothorax, and is often secondary to pneumonia. A pneumothorax occurs when air enters the pleural cavity.

CHAPTER 7
The Cardiovascular System (MCQs)

7.1. The left atrium of the heart receives oxygenated blood from the:

- A) Pulmonary veins
- B) Inferior vena cava (IVC)
- C) Superior vena cava (SVC)
- D) Pulmonary trunk

7.2. The arch of the aorta typically gives rise to three arterial branches. Which of the following vessels is **not** a branch of the aortic arch?

- A) Left common carotid artery
- B) Left subclavian artery
- C) Right coronary artery
- D) Brachiocephalic trunk

7.3. A number of functional and anatomical differences exist between arteries and veins. Which of the following statements is **false** with regard to the significant distinctions between these two blood vessels?

- A) Arteries carry oxygenated blood, under high pressure, away from the heart to tissues and organs while veins return deoxygenated blood, under low pressure, to the heart
- B) Veins contain valves to prevent the back-flow of blood
- C) Arteries have a thin tunica media and veins have a thick tunica media, due to pressure differences between the two blood vessels
- D) Arteries appear pulsatile and are non-compressible on a vascular ultrasound, while veins appear non-pulsatile and are easily compressible

7.4. The wall of the heart is composed of three basic layers. Which of these layers is the **thickest**?

- A) Endocardium
- B) Myocardium
- C) Epicardium
- D) Tunica adventitia

7.5. Which of the following statements is **false** with regard to the four heart valves and their location?

A) The aortic valve is located between the right ventricle and the aorta
B) The mitral valve is located between the left atrium and left ventricle
C) The tricuspid valve is located between the right atrium and right ventricle
D) The pulmonary valve is located between the right ventricle and pulmonary trunk

7.6. The sinoatrial node (SA node), or primary pacemaker of the heart, is located in the wall of which chamber?

A) Left atrium
B) Right atrium
C) Left ventricle
D) Right ventricle

7.7. Which of the following statements is **true** with regard to the similarities and differences between cardiac muscle and skeletal muscle?

A) Striations are present in skeletal muscle, but not cardiac muscle
B) Cardiac muscle is under voluntary control by the somatic motor system, while skeletal muscle is controlled involuntarily by the autonomic nervous system and the endocrine system
C) Intercalated disks are specialised cell-cell junctions that are found in cardiac muscle, but not skeletal muscle
D) All of the above

7.8. Cardiac output (CO) describes the volume of blood ejected from the heart in one minute, and is calculated as follows:

Cardiac Output (CO) = Heart Rate (HR) x Stroke Volume (SV)

Based on the equation above, cardiac output will **increase** if:

A) Heart rate is decreased
B) Heart rate is increased
C) Stroke volume is decreased
D) Stroke volume remains the same

CHAPTER 7: The Cardiovascular System (MCQs)

7.9. Which of the following hormones will cause a **decrease** in blood pressure (BP)?

A) Angiotensin II
B) Atrial natriuretic peptide (ANP)
C) Antidiuretic hormone (ADH)
D) Aldosterone

7.10. Capillaries are divided into three types based on the structure of their endothelial layer: continuous, fenestrated, and sinusoid. Fenestrated capillaries are typically located in the:

A) Liver
B) Spleen
C) Nervous system
D) Kidney glomeruli

7.11. Which of the following heart diseases is **congenital** (present from birth)?

A) Tetralogy of Fallot (ToF)
B) Atrial fibrillation (AF)
C) Congestive heart failure (CHF)
D) Complete heart block

7.12. Which of the following is a **non-modifiable** risk factor for the development and progression of atherosclerosis?

A) Family history
B) Smoking
C) Hyperlipidaemia
D) Hypertension

7.13. Virchow's triad describes three risk factors that predispose an individual to thrombus formation. Which of the following is **not** a component of Virchow's triad?

A) Hypercoagulability
B) Endothelial injury
C) Blood flow stasis
D) Vasodilation

7.14. The resting heart rate (RHR) of an elite athlete is most likely to fall within which of the following ranges:

- A) 30-40 beats/min
- B) 50-60 beats/min
- C) 70-80 bears/min
- D) 90-100 beats/min

7.15. Hypertension is clinically defined as a systolic and/or diastolic blood pressure level consistently at or above:

- A) 120/70 mmHg
- B) 130/80 mmHg
- C) 140/90 mmHg
- D) 150/100 mmHg

7.16. Which of the following terms is used to describe the force per unit area exerted by circulating blood on the vessel wall?

- A) Heart rate (HR)
- B) Blood pressure (BP)
- C) Blood velocity (V)
- D) Blood flow (Q)

7.17. An electrocardiogram (ECG) is a diagnostic tool used to view the electrical activity of the heart. Which of the following statements is **false** with regard to the different components of an ECG?

- A) The P-wave denotes atrial depolarization and the QRS complex represents ventricular depolarization
- B) The T-wave denotes ventricular repolarization
- C) The PR interval represents the time delay between atrial and ventricular depolarization, which occurs at the atrioventricular (AV) node
- D) The first negative (downward) deflection on an ECG after the P-wave is the R-wave

CHAPTER 7: The Cardiovascular System (MCQs)

7.18. The foetal circulation contains three shunts that allow blood to bypass the foetal lungs and liver during development. Which of the following statements is **false** with regard to the physiologic shunts present in the foetal circulatory system?

A) The umbilical vein carries oxygenated blood from the placenta to the liver
B) The ductus venosus is a shunt that allows blood to bypass the liver
C) The foramen ovale allows blood to bypass the lungs and pass directly from the left atrium to the right atrium
D) The ductus arteriosus provides a shunt between the pulmonary trunk and the aorta

7.19. Which of the following statements is **false** with regard to the circulatory changes that occur following birth?

A) Termination of the umbilical circulation causes the ductus venosus to close and degenerate
B) The ligamentum venosum is the adult remnant of the ductus venosus
C) Functional closure of the foramen ovale occurs in association with the neonate's first breath at birth
D) The remnant of the foramen ovale in the adult heart is known as the septum secundum

7.20. The ductus arteriosus typically closes spontaneously at birth, if it fails to do so then continual shunting of blood from the aorta to the pulmonary artery will occur. Which of the following statements is **true** with regard to the presence of a patent ductus arteriosus after birth?

A) The ductus arteriosus typically closes at birth due to increasing oxygen tension in the aorta and a decrease in circulating prostaglandins
B) A patent ductus arteriosus is treated with prostaglandin inhibitors
C) It can lead to pulmonary hypertension, right ventricular hypertrophy and eventually heart failure
D) All of the above

7.21. Ventricular septal defects (VSDs) are the most common form of congenital heart defect. Which of the following statements is **false** with regard to the size, location and haemodynamic effect of these congenital malformations?

A) The defect can affect the muscular or membranous part of the interventricular septum (IVS)
B) Ventricular septal defects allow blood to shunt from the left to the right-hand side of the heart
C) Small defects often close spontaneously
D) Large defects can progress to pulmonary hypertension and hypertrophy of the left ventricle

7.22. There are two main types of valvular heart disease: stenosis and regurgitation. Which of the following statements is **false** with regard to these valvular abnormalities?

A) Valvular stenosis is marked by failure of a valve to close completely, while valvular regurgitation is marked by failure of a valve to open completely
B) Valvular stenosis leads to pressure overload of the heart
C) Valvular regurgitation leads to volume overload of the heart
D) Regurgitant valves are also called incompetent or insufficient valves

7.23 Which of the following thrombotic disorders is **not** an example of arterial thrombosis?

A) Myocardial infarction (MI)
B) Atrial fibrillation (AF)
C) Pulmonary embolism (PE)
D) Cerebral infarction

7.24. The structural response to aortic stenosis (AS) is an increase in the mass and relative wall thickness of the left ventricle of the heart. This is an example of which type of adaptive response?

A) Atrophy
B) Hyperplasia
C) Hypertrophy
D) Metaplasia

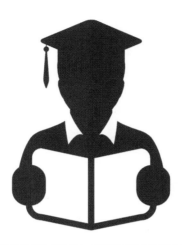

CHAPTER 7

The Cardiovascular System (MCQs)

Answers and Detailed Solutions

The difficulty rating for each question (Easy, Moderate or Hard) can be found in parentheses next to the correct answer.

7.1. A (Easy)

The human heart pumps around 5 litres of blood per minute. Deoxygenated blood from the upper and lower body regions is collected through the superior vena cava (SVC) and inferior vena cava (IVC) respectively, and drains into the right atrium of the heart. It then travels through the tricuspid valve into the right ventricle, and is pumped through the pulmonary trunk (which divides into a left and right pulmonary artery) into the lungs for oxygenation. Once blood has been oxygenated in the lungs it returns to the left atrium of the heart via the four pulmonary veins. It then passes via the mitral valve into the left ventricle, which pumps it through the aortic valve into the aorta and to the rest of the body.

7.2. C (Easy)

There are three blood vessels that typically branch off the arch of the aorta. On the left-hand side, the left common carotid artery and left subclavian artery come directly off the aortic arch. On the right-hand side, the brachiocephalic trunk runs a short distance superiorly and then bifurcates into the right subclavian artery and the right common carotid artery. In contrast, the right coronary artery (RCA) branches from the ascending aorta. The left and right coronary arteries (LCA and RCA) are the only branches to come from the ascending aorta.

7.3. C (Moderate)

There are a number of significant anatomical, functional and structural differences between arteries and veins. Arteries carry oxygenated blood, under high pressure, away from the heart to tissues and organs, while veins return deoxygenated blood, under low pressure, to the heart. As a result of this pressure difference, arteries have a thick tunica media and veins have a thin tunica media. Arteries appear pulsatile and are non-compressible on a vascular ultrasound, while veins appear non-pulsatile and are easily compressible. In addition, veins contain valves to prevent the back-flow of blood.

7.4. B (Easy)

The myocardium (middle layer) is the thickest of the three layers of the heart, as it consists of cardiac muscle. This muscular layer is responsible for the contractile function of the atria and ventricles. The inner lining of the heart is called the endocardium, while the outermost layer is the epicardium. The latter is equivalent to the tunica adventitia (outer layer) of the vasculature in the arterial and venous system.

7.5. A (Easy)

The aortic valve is located between the left ventricle and the aorta, while the pulmonary valve is located between the right ventricle and pulmonary trunk (which divides into a left and right pulmonary artery). Likewise, the mitral valve is located between the left atrium and left ventricle, and the tricuspid valve is located between the right atrium and right ventricle.

7.6. B (Easy)

The sinoatrial node (SA node), or primary pacemaker of the heart, is located in the posterior wall of the right atrium, near to the opening of the superior vena cava (SVC). Each cardiac cycle is initiated by this small mass of specialised cells. The cardiac action potential originates in the sinoatrial node, and then propagates to the secondary pacemaker, the atrioventricular node (AV node), via internodal pathways in the atria.

7.7. C (Hard)

Cardiac muscle is a specialised form of skeletal muscle and, as such, also contains striations. Cardiac muscle is controlled involuntarily by the autonomic nervous system and the endocrine system, while skeletal muscle is under voluntary or conscious control by the somatic motor system (somatic nervous system). Moreover, intercalated disks are specialised cell-cell junctions that are found in cardiac muscle, but not skeletal muscle.

7.8. B (Moderate)

Cardiac output (CO) is dependant upon two factors: heart rate (HR) and stroke volume (SV). Stroke volume is the volume of blood ejected from the heart in one ventricular contraction. As such, it refers to the difference between end-diastolic volume (EDV, the volume of blood in the ventricle prior to contraction) and end-systolic volume (ESV, the volume of blood that remains in the ventricle after contraction), and is calculated using the following equation:

Stroke Volume (SV) = End-diastolic volume (EDV) − End-systolic volume (ESV)

Heart rate (HR) is described as the number of heart beats per unit of time. Along these lines, cardiac output will increase if heart rate or stroke volume is increased.

7.9. B (Hard)

Atrial natriuretic peptide (ANP) will cause blood volume to decrease and thus lead to a fall in blood pressure (BP). In contrast, aldosterone and antidiuretic hormone (ADH) or vasopressin, will cause blood volume to increase and thus lead to a rise in blood pressure. Angiotensin II stimulates the release of aldosterone and antidiuretic hormone (ADH), and also causes vasoconstriction, which will likewise lead to an increase in blood pressure.

7.10. D (Moderate)

Kidney glomeruli consist of fenestrated capillaries, and thus contain numerous fenestrations (small windows) or pores in the endothelium, which enhance permeability in the kidney. The small intestine and endocrine glands also contain fenestrated capillaries. Sinusoid (discontinuous) capillaries are typically found in areas capable of haematopoiesis, such as the liver, spleen and bone marrow. Continuous capillaries can be located in the nervous system, as well as in muscle and the lungs. These capillaries contain tight non-permeable junctions between endothelial cells.

7.11. A (Moderate)

Tetralogy of Fallot (ToF) or Fallot's tetralogy is a cyanotic congenital heart disease, characterised by a collection of four malformations. These abnormalities are all caused by unequal division of the truncus arteriosus, due to anterior displacement of the aorticopulmonary septum during embryogenesis. It is marked by the following four cardiac defects: pulmonary stenosis, ventricular septal defect (VSD), an overriding aorta that is shifted to the right and right ventricular hypertrophy due to increased pressure on the right-hand side of the heart. This constellation of abnormalities results in cyanosis, due to right to left shunt.

7.12. A (Easy)

Family history is a non-modifiable risk factor for the development and progression of atherosclerosis, as it is inherited. Conversely, hyperlipidaemia (high serum cholesterol), hypertension (high blood pressure) and smoking are modifiable risk factors for the development and progression of atherosclerosis, as they can be altered by lifestyle factors (behaviour and diet).

7.13. D (Hard)

Patients are at increased risk of venous thrombosis, according to Virchow's triad, if they exhibit one or more of the following predisposing factors: circulatory or blood flow stasis, endothelial dysfunction or injury, and their blood is in a hypercoagulable state. Vasodilation is not a component of Virchow's triad.

7.14. A (Moderate)

Normal resting heart rate (RHR) is around 60-100 beats/min. In contrast, elite athletes are likely to have a resting heart rate of 30-40 beats/min or lower. These normal ranges can, of course, be affected by environmental factors such as altitude and temperature. Furthermore, in a phenomenon known as anticipatory response (or rise), heart rate (HR) increases above resting heart rate prior to the start of exercise.

7.15. C (Easy)

Hypertension (high blood pressure) is a major risk factor for myocardial infarction (MI), heart failure and kidney disease. It is clinically defined as a systolic and/or diastolic blood pressure level consistently at or above 140/90 mmHg. A normal blood pressure is clinically defined as a blood pressure level consistently around 120-135/70-85 mmHg. Clinicians aim for tighter blood pressure control in patients with diabetes and, as such, aim for a blood pressure level consistently below 130/80 mmHg. A blood pressure level consistently above 180/120 mmHg, is referred to as malignant hypertension and is often accompanied by signs and symptoms of organ damage. Malignant hypertension requires urgent therapeutic intervention in order to preserve organ function.

[The criteria for blood pressure treatment changes year on year, as new guidelines are produced, therefore while the information above does correlate with current treatment targets at the time of publication, please be aware that these thresholds are subject to change.]

7.16. B (Moderate)

Heart rate (HR) is described as the number of heart beats per unit of time. Blood pressure (BP) is the force per unit area exerted by circulating blood on the vessel wall. Blood velocity (V) is the distance travelled per unit of time by individual cells within the blood. Blood flow (Q) is the volume per unit time of blood through a vessel.

7.17. D (Hard)

On an electrocardiogram (ECG), the P-wave denotes atrial depolarization, while the QRS complex represents ventricular depolarization. The T-wave denotes ventricular repolarization and the PR interval represents the time delay between atrial and ventricular depolarization, which occurs at the atrioventricular node (AV node). Furthermore, the first negative (downward) deflection on an ECG after the P-wave is the Q-wave, while the first positive (upward) deflection is the R-wave.

7.18. C (Hard)

All of the changes that occur in the foetal circulation are due to the fact that oxygenated blood comes from the placenta, as opposed to the lungs. The umbilical vein carries oxygenated blood from the placenta into the foetal circulation. Once the umbilical vein has reached the liver, a small amount of blood will enter the liver and the rest will bypass the liver via the ductus venosus and enter the inferior vena cava (IVC). The inferior vena cava then enters the right atrium. The majority of this oxygenated blood will bypass the lungs and pass directly from the **right** atrium to the **left** atrium, via the foramen ovale. In addition, the ductus arteriosus provides a shunt between the pulmonary trunk and the aorta, and reduces the oxygenation of the blood in the aorta.

7.19. D (Hard)

When the neonate is delivered, the umbilical vessels that connect to the placenta are clipped off. This termination of the umbilical circulation causes the ductus venosus to close and degenerate, leaving the ligamentum venosum - the adult remnant of the ductus venosus. Functional closure of the foraman ovale occurs in association with the neonate's first breath at birth. The neonate's first breath opens up the pulmonary circulation, and leads to pressure changes in the atria. Fluid moves out of the lungs and blood return to the heart increases through the pulmonary veins. This leads to an increase in pressure in the left atrium, which pushes the septum primum against the septum secundum, closing the foramen ovale. The remnant of the foramen ovale in the adult heart is known as the fossa ovalis (not the septum secundum).

7.20. D (Hard)

The ductus arteriosus, situated between the pulmonary trunk and the aorta, normally closes at birth in response to increasing oxygen tension in the aorta and a decrease in circulating prostaglandins. The ductus arteriosus contains contractile cells that will contract in response to an increase in oxygen tension and a decrease in prostaglandins. Prior to birth, the pressure in the heart is higher on the right-hand side, which means that foetal blood is pumped from the pulmonary trunk into the aorta, through a patent ductus arteriosus. After birth, however, the pressure is higher on the left-hand side of the heart, and this means, if the ductus arteriosus fails to close, that blood is pumped from the aorta into the pulmonary trunk. This is problematic as blood that is already oxygenated is being pushed back into the lungs. As such, the workload of the pulmonary circulation is increased, which can lead to pulmonary hypertension. The resultant increase in pressure on the right-hand side of the heart, due to changes in the pulmonary circulation, can also lead to hypertrophy of the right ventricle. The combination of pulmonary hypertension and ventricular hypertrophy over a sustained period of time will eventually result in heart failure, which is potentially fatal. Infants with a patent ductus arteriousus will thus be treated with prostaglandin inhibitors in an effort to close the structure, and prevent these complications.

7.21. D (Hard)

Ventricular septal defects (VSDs) are the most common form of congenital heart defect, and are often associated with other congenital malformations. Along these lines, VSDs are classically associated with Down's syndrome. The defect can affect the muscular or membranous part of the interventricular septum (IVS), although around 90% of cases involve the membranous septum. VSDs allow blood to shunt from the left to the right-hand side of the heart. This puts extra stress on the right side of the heart and can lead to hypertrophy of the right ventricle. Large defects can therefore progress to pulmonary hypertension and hypertrophy of the right (not the left) ventricle, while small defects often close spontaneously.

7.22. A (Moderate)

Valvular stenosis is marked by failure of a valve to open completely, while valvular regurgitation is marked by failure of a valve to close completely. The former impedes forward flow, while the latter facilitates reverse flow. Along these lines, valvular stenosis leads to pressure overload of the heart, and valvular regurgitation leads to volume overload of the heart. Valvular regurgitation is also called incompetence or "insufficiency".

7.23. C (Easy)

Thrombosis involves the formation of a blood clot inside a vessel, which obstructs circulation. There are two main types of thrombus: venous and arterial. Myocardial infarction (MI), atrial fibrillation (AF) and cerebral infarction or stroke are all examples of arterial thrombosis. In contrast, pulmonary embolism (PE) and deep vein thrombosis (DVT), are examples of venous thrombosis. Arterial thrombi are typically platelet rich, while venous thrombi are typically rich in erythrocytes and fibrin.

7.24. C (Moderate)

Hypertrophy is common in cardiac muscle and describes an increase in the size of existing cells, as well as an increase in functional capacity. Aortic stenosis (AS) occurs when the aortic valve does not open properly. This results in left ventricular hypertrophy, as the systolic pressure in the left ventricle needs to be high in order to generate the same amount of flow across the stenotic valve. Atrophy describes a decrease in cell size and number, while hyperplasia refers to an increase in cell number due to cell division. Moreover, metaplasia describes the transformation of one differentiated cell type into another one.

CHAPTER 8
The Gastrointestinal System (MCQs)

8.1. The gastrointestinal (GI) tract can be divided into three sections: the foregut, midgut and hindgut. Which of these regions extends from the second half of the duodenum to two-thirds of the way along the transverse colon?

A) Foregut
B) Midgut
C) Hindgut
D) None of the above

8.2. The blood supply to the gastrointestinal tract is derived from three branches of the abdominal aorta: the coeliac artery, superior mesenteric artery (SMA) and inferior mesenteric artery (IMA). Which of the following statements is **false** with regard to the arterial supply to the gastrointestinal tract?

A) The coeliac artery supplies foregut structures
B) The superior mesenteric artery supplies midgut structures
C) The inferior mesenteric artery supplies hindgut structures
D) The marginal artery of the colon connects branches of the superior mesenteric artery with the coeliac artery

The following **six** questions concern the clinical anatomy of the abdomen, and the points of reference and landmarks used by clinicians for abdominal examination.

During clinical examination, the abdominal cavity is divided into nine distinct regions or sections. This is largely for descriptive purposes, and is used to identify the location of specific abdominal organs.

These nine regions can be seen on the following diagram:

Right Hypochondrium	Epigastrium	Left Hypochondrium
Right Lumbar	Umbilical	Left Lumbar
Right Iliac	Hypogastric (Suprapubic)	Left Iliac

[The abdominal cavity stretches from the diaphragm superiorly to the pelvic inlet inferiorly.]

8.3. The ascending colon is located in which of the following abdominal regions?

   A) Right Hypochondrium
   B) Right Lumbar
   C) Right Iliac
   D) Umbilical

8.4. The liver is located in which of the following abdominal regions?

   A) Epigastrium and Left Hypochondrium
   B) Umbilical and Left Lumbar
   C) Right Hypochondrium and Epigastrium
   D) Right Lumbar and Umbilical

8.5. The sigmoid colon is located in which of the following abdominal regions?

   A) Right Iliac
   B) Left Iliac
   C) Umbilical
   D) Hypogastrium

For the purposes of abdominal examination, the abdomen is also classically divided into four quadrants. This four-quadrant system is defined by horizontal and vertical planes that intersect at the umbilicus.

These four quadrants can be seen on the following diagram:

Right Upper Quadrant (RUQ)	Left Upper Quadrant (LUQ)
Right Lower Quadrant (RLQ)	Left Lower Quadrant (LLQ)

8.6. The gall bladder is located in which of the following abdominal quadrants?

   A) Right Upper Quadrant
   B) Left Upper Quadrant
   C) Right Lower Quadrant
   D) Left Lower Quadrant

CHAPTER 8: The Gastrointestinal System (MCQs)

8.7. The caecum and appendix are located in which of the following abdominal quadrants?

A) Right Upper Quadrant
B) Left Upper Quadrant
C) Right Lower Quadrant
D) Left Lower Quadrant

8.8. The spleen is located in which of the following abdominal quadrants?

A) Right Upper Quadrant
B) Left Upper Quadrant
C) Right Lower Quadrant
D) Left Lower Quadrant

8.9. Which of the following abdominal organs is protected by the thoracic cage (rib cage)?

A) Liver
B) Spleen
C) Kidneys (superior pole)
D) All of the above

8.10. There are three pairs of major salivary glands: parotid, submandibular and sublingual. Which of the following statements is **true** with regard to the structure and function of these large glands?

A) The submandibular is the largest salivary gland
B) The sublingual gland is the main source of lysozyme and lactoperoxidase
C) The parotid gland is the main source of salivary amylase and proline rich-proteins
D) The submandibular gland produces a predominately serous secretion

8.11. Which of the following regions of the stomach are primarily involved in **acid** secretion?

A) Cardia
B) Fundus and Body
C) Antrum
D) Pylorus

8.12. Which of the following small bowel motility patterns is defined as a set of rhythmic, wave-like muscular contractions that transport food along the length of the gastrointestinal tract?

A) Peristalsis
B) Segmentation
C) Migrating Motor Complex (MMC)
D) None of the above

8.13. Which of the following statements is **false** with regard to the structure and function of the pancreas?

A) The pancreas has both endocrine and exocrine functions
B) It is a non-encapsulated, retroperitoneal structure
C) The pancreas secretes a range of digestive hormones in an acidic fluid
D) Proteolytic enzymes from the pancreas are secreted as inactive proenzymes or zymogens

8.14. The irreversible loss of **endocrine** tissue in chronic pancreatitis will lead to a reduction in which of the following pancreatic secretions?

A) Trypsin
B) Amylase
C) Insulin
D) Elastase

8.15. Which of the following pancreatic enzymes is involved in the chemical digestion of fat?

A) Trypsinogen
B) Chymotrypsinogen
C) Pancreatic lipase
D) Ribonuclease

8.16. The islets of Langerhans in the pancreas are composed of multiple functional cell types, each of which secretes a different peptide hormone. Insulin is produced by which of the following cell types?

A) β cells
B) α cells
C) δ cells
D) F or PP cells

8.17. Which of the following metabolic processes helps to maintain blood glucose levels during fasting?

A) Glycogenolysis
B) Gluconeogenesis
C) A and B
D) None of the above

8.18. Inflammatory bowel disease (IBD) is a chronic condition, characterised by inflammation of the tissue lining the gastrointestinal tract, and of which there are two main types: Crohn's disease (CD) and ulcerative colitis (UC). Which of the following is a complication of Crohn's disease but **not** ulcerative colitis?

A) Haemorrhage
B) Fistula formation
C) Toxic megacolon
D) Carcinoma

8.19. Which of the following is a **not** a presenting sign or symptom of gastrointestinal disease?

A) Dysphagia
B) Nausea and vomiting
C) Haemoptysis
D) Rectal bleeding

8.20. Which of the following statements is **false** with regard to the major functions and motility patterns in the large bowel (large intestine)?

A) The absorption of water and electrolytes is a key function of the large bowel
B) Colonic bacteria digest fibre and other unused nutrients
C) Haustration describes a mixing movement, in which the slow contraction of circular muscle squeezes the contents of the large bowel
D) Around 1-3 times a minute, the propulsion of stool along the colon and towards the rectum occurs in what is known as a mass movement

8.21. Individuals with a body mass index (BMI) of 30 or higher, are at increased risk of:

A) Coronary heart disease (CHD)
B) Osteoarthritis
C) Type II diabetes mellitus
D) All of the above

8.22. Which of the following is **not** a function of the liver?

A) The production and secretion of bile
B) Drug metabolism
C) Erythropoiesis
D) Protein synthesis

8.23. Which of the following vitamins is **not** fat-soluble?

A) A
B) C
C) E
D) K

8.24. Severe vitamin A deficiency can lead to:

A) Xerophthalmia
B) Beri beri
C) Pellagra
D) Bleeding disorders

CHAPTER 8

The Gastrointestinal System (MCQs)

Answers and Detailed Solutions

The difficulty rating for each question (Easy, Moderate or Hard) can be found in parentheses next to the correct answer.

8.1. B (Moderate)

The midgut extends from the second half of the duodenum through the jejunum, ilium, appendix, caecum and ascending colon to two-thirds of the way along the transverse colon. The hindgut extends along the remainder of the transverse colon, through the descending colon and sigmoid colon to the rectum. The foregut extends from the mouth to the first half of the duodenum.

8.2. D (Hard)

The coeliac artery supplies foregut structures (the abdominal oesophagus, spleen, stomach, liver, gall bladder, pancreas and the first half of the duodenum). The superior mesenteric artery (SMA) supplies midgut structures (the second half of the duodenum, jejunum, ileum, appendix, caecum, ascending colon, hepatic flexure and the proximal two-thirds of the transverse colon). The inferior mesenteric artery (IMA) supplies hindgut structures (the distal one-third of the transverse colon, splenic flexure, descending colon, sigmoid colon and the rectum). In addition, the marginal artery of the colon, also known as the marginal artery of Drummond, connects branches of the superior mesenteric artery with the inferior mesenteric artery.

8.3. B (Moderate)

The ascending colon is located in the middle zone of the abdomen, in the right lumber (or right flank) region. The right kidney and part of the small intestine are also located in this region. The descending colon is located in the left lumbar region.

8.4. C (Moderate)

The liver is located in the upper zone of the abdomen, and extends over multiple regions. To this end, it is found in both the right hypochondrium region and the epigastric region.

8.5. B (Moderate)

The sigmoid colon and part of the small intestine are located in the left iliac region, while the terminal ileum, appendix and caecum are located in the right iliac region.

8.6. A (Easy)

The gall bladder is located in the right upper quadrant (RUQ). The liver, hepatic flexure of the colon, portions of the ascending and transverse colon, right kidney and the head of the pancreas are also located in this quadrant.

8.7. C (Easy)

The caecum and appendix are located in the right lower quadrant (RLQ). The lower pole of the right kidney, a portion of the ascending colon, reproductive organs (such as the right ovary in females and the right spermatic cord in males) and the right ureter are also located in this quadrant.

8.8. B (Easy)

The spleen is located in the left upper quadrant (LUQ). The body of the pancreas, splenic flexure of the colon, portions of the descending and transverse colon, left kidney, the left lobe of the liver and the stomach are also located in this quadrant.

8.9. D (Easy)

The thoracic cage (rib cage) encloses and protects a number of vital, life-sustaining organs. These include the heart and lungs, as well as various abdominal organs. Along these lines, the liver, spleen, superior pole of the kidneys and cardia and fundus of the stomach are all protected by the thoracic cage. For this reason, the liver, spleen and superior pole of the kidneys are not usually palpable during organ specific palpation in healthy individuals, unless they are extremely thin.

8.10. C (Hard)

The parotid (not the submandibular) gland is the largest salivary gland. The submandibular (not the sublingual) gland is the main source of lysozyme and lactoperoxidase. The sublingual gland is the main source of lingual lipase. Likewise, the parotid gland is the main source of salivary amylase and proline rich-proteins. The submandibular gland produces a mixture of mucous and serous secretions, while the parotid gland produces a predominately serous secretion and the sublingual gland produces a predominantly mucous secretion.

8.11. B (Hard)

The stomach churns and stores food, and produces acid to facilitate digestion and the chemical breakdown process. Acid, along with intrinsic factor (IF), pepsinogens, lipase, mucus and bicarbonate (HCO_3^-), is predominantly secreted in the fundus and body of the stomach. Mucus and bicarbonate are the dominant secretions in the cardia, as well as in the antrum and pylorus.

8.12. A (Moderate)

Peristalsis is defined as a set of rhythmic, wave-like muscular contractions that transport food along the length of the gastrointestinal tract. Segmentation describes the alternate contraction of neighbouring segments of circular muscle, in order to mix the contents of the lumen. In contrast to peristalsis and segmentation, the migrating motor complex (MMC) occurs when the gut is relatively empty. It is generated by the hormone motilin, and consists of a series of slow but strong peristaltic waves that start in the stomach and sweep down through the small intestine. These cleansing waves help to safeguard against reflux, keep the small intestine clean and limit bacterial growth in the small bowel.

8.13. C (Moderate)

The pancreas is a non-encapsulated, retroperitoneal structure, located deep in the abdomen and situated posterior to the stomach. This elongated gland secretes a range of digestive hormones in an alkaline (not an acidic) fluid. The organ also has both endocrine and exocrine functions.

The endocrine tissue secretes peptide hormones (such as insulin and glucagon) into the blood, while exocrine tissue produces digestive enzymes (such as trypsin, lipase and elastase), which assist in the chemical breakdown of food. With regard to the latter, it is important to note that proteolytic enzymes are secreted as inactive proenzymes or zymogens, in order to prevent auto-digestion of the pancreas.

8.14. C (Hard)

Exocrine tissue, which comprises the vast majority of the pancreas (around 85%), secretes digestive enzymes such as amylase, elastase and trypsin. By contrast, peptide hormones, like insulin, are secreted directly into the bloodstream by endocrine tissue. The irreversible destruction of exocrine tissue seen in chronic pancreatitis is followed by the destruction of endocrine tissue. This loss of endocrine tissue, however, is a late feature of chronic pancreatitis, as the islets of Langerhans are relatively resistant to destruction.

[Strictly speaking, as both exocrine and endocrine tissue are lost in chronic pancreatitis, all of the pancreatic secretions in this question would reduce. This question, however, is specifically testing your ability to differentiate between endocrine and exocrine function.]

8.15. C (Easy)

Trypsinogen and chymotrypsinogen are endoproteases. Along with exoproteases, such as procarboxypeptidases A and B, these enzymes hydrolyse the peptide bonds in proteins and polypeptides, at the middle and end of the chain respectively. Pancreatic lipase, along with nonspecific esterase and prophospholipase A2, is involved in the chemical digestion of fat. Moreover, ribonuclease is involved in the digestion of different types of RNA.

8.16. A (Moderate)

In the islets of Langerhans, β cells produce insulin, primarily in response to blood glucose levels but also other stimuli. Likewise, α cells produce glucagon, which antagonises the effects of insulin. In addition, δ cells secrete somatostatin and F or PP cells secrete pancreatic polypeptide (PP).

These different cell types cannot be distinguished by routine haematoxylin and eosin (H&E) staining, therefore immunocytochemistry is used to differentiate between them.

8.17. C (Moderate)

The breakdown of stored glycogen to glucose is known as glycogenolysis, and the *de novo* synthesis of glucose from a variety of non-glucose substrates (amino acids, lactate, pyruvate and glycerol) is known as gluconeogenesis. Both of these metabolic processes help to maintain blood glucose levels during fasting.

8.18. B (Hard)

The risk of carcinoma of the large bowel is equivalent in ulcerative colitis (UC) and Crohn's disease (CD). Fistulas are seen in Crohn's disease as the inflammation is transmural, and this can lead to the emergence of deep fissuring ulcers, which extend all the way through the bowel wall and become adherent to other structures, resulting in fistula formation between the bowel and other structures (e.g. the abdominal wall). In contrast, fistulas are not seen in ulcerative colitis as the inflammation is limited to the mucosa and submucosa. Severe inflammation can also lead to dilatation of the colon (toxic megacolon) in both ulcerative colitis and Crohn's disease, although it is much more common in the former. Similarly, haemorrhage is a complication of both ulcerative colitis and Crohn's disease, due to ulceration in the bowel and erosion into the blood vessels. In addition, the presence of granulomas is a classic microscopic feature of Crohn's disease, seen in around 50-60% of cases.

8.19. C (Hard)

Nausea and vomiting, rectal bleeding and dysphagia are all presenting features of gastrointestinal disease. Nausea and vomiting is a non-specific symptom in isolation; if it is associated with other symptoms, however, there are a number of possible diagnoses. When associated with diarrhoea it is likely to be gastroenteritis. Similarly, when associated with abdominal pain it could be a presenting feature of pancreatitis or peptic ulcer disease

(PUD). Likewise, in association with abdominal pain and bloating, it could be due to obstruction of the gastrointestinal tract. In like manner, nausea and vomiting in association with weight loss could be a result of gastric outflow obstruction. Rectal bleeding is commonly caused by an anal fissure or haemorrhoids. It can also be seen in inflammatory bowel disease (IBD), colorectal cancer and as a complication of diverticular disease. The development of dysphagia (difficulty swallowing) is an alarm symptom for oesophageal cancer. Dysphagia can also be caused by the oesophageal motility disorder, achalasia. In contrast, haemoptysis, the coughing up of blood, is a symptom associated with the respiratory system.

8.20. D (Hard)

There are two key motility patterns in the large bowel: haustration and mass movement. The former describes a mixing movement, in which the slow contraction of circular muscle squeezes the contents of the large bowel. The latter, occurs around 1-3 times a day (not a minute!), and involves the propulsion of stool along the colon and towards the rectum. With regard to function, the absorption of water and electrolytes is a key function of the large bowel. In like manner, colonic bacteria digest fibre and other unused nutrients in the large bowel. Bacteria digest the amino acids Cysteine (Cys) and Methionine (Met), for instance, and they are converted to hydrogen sulphide. Similarly, fibre is digested by bacteria in the colon, and this produces short chain fatty acids such as butyric acid, as well as methane and hydrogen.

8.21. D (Easy)

Individuals with a body mass index (BMI) of 30 or higher, are classified as obese and thus at increased risk of a number of diseases. These include type II diabetes mellitus, due to insulin resistance and coronary heart disease (CHD) due to the increased strain that is placed upon their cardiovascular system. Those who are obese are also at increased risk of developing osteoarthritis, as the extra weight that they are carrying places considerable pressure on their joints.

8.22. C (Easy)

The production and secretion of bile is a major function of the liver. The gall bladder is then involved in the storage and concentration of bile. Likewise, drug metabolism and protein synthesis are functions of the liver, along with the metabolism and homeostasis of iron, and the storage and metabolism of vitamins and nutrients. Erythropoiesis (the production of red blood cells), however, occurs in the kidneys, not the liver.

8.23. B (Easy)

The fat-soluble vitamins are A, D, E and K. These four vitamins closely follow the standard pathways of lipid absorption and, as such, can dissolve in lipid droplets, micelles and chylomicrons. Deficiency in these vitamins can result if fat absorption is impaired. In contrast, vitamin C (ascorbic acid) is a water-soluble vitamin.

8.24. A (Hard)

Xerophthalmia is an ocular consequence of severe vitamin A deficiency. This is marked by very dry eyes (due to dryness of the cornea and conjunctiva), and can lead to night blindness (the inability to see in dim light). Vitamin K is involved in the development of blood clotting factors and, as such, deficiencies in vitamin K can lead to abnormal clotting and bleeding disorders. Pellagra (meaning 'dry skin' in Italian) is seen in niacin (vitamin B_3) deficiency, and is characterised by the classical triad of dermatitis, diarrhoea and dementia. Beri beri is linked to prolonged thiamine (vitamin B_1) deficiency, and consists of three different types. These include, wet beri beri, which affects the cardiovascular system, dry beri beri, which affects the nervous system and has neuritic manifestations, and infantile beri beri, which is observed in breast-fed infants whose mothers are thiamine deficient.

CHAPTER 9
The Renal System (MCQs)

9.1. Which of the following statements is **false** with regard to the anatomy of the kidneys?

A) They are located either side of the vertebral column between the last thoracic vertebra (T12) and the third lumbar vertebra (L3)
B) They are retroperitoneal structures
C) Healthy kidneys are approximately 10-11cm in length
D) The right kidney lies at a higher level than the left kidney

9.2. Nephrons are the microscopic, functional units of the kidney, in which urine formation takes place through a complex, three-step process of filtration, reabsorption and secretion. Which of the following statements is **false** with regard to the structural components of the renal nephron and its microvasculature?

A) The renal tubule consists of several segments. Nearest to the glomerulus is the proximal tubule, followed by the loop of Henle and the distal convoluted tubule, which connects to the collecting duct system
B) The glomerulus is a knot of capillaries located in the Bowman's capsule, within the renal medulla
C) The afferent arteriole, a branch of the interlobular artery, enters the Bowman's capsule and branches into the glomerular capillaries
D) The distal end of the glomerular capillaries reunite to form an efferent arteriole, which leaves the glomerulus

9.3. The two adrenal or suprarenal glands are endocrine organs, situated on the upper pole of the kidneys. Each of these structures receives a rich and delicate blood supply from three main groups of arteries: the superior, middle and inferior suprarenal arteries. Which of these blood vessels originates from the **left** renal artery?

A) Left superior suprarenal artery
B) Right superior suprarenal artery
C) Left middle suprarenal artery
D) Left inferior suprarenal artery

9.4. Which of the following organs lies in contact with the anterior surface of the **right** kidney?

A) Spleen
B) Stomach
C) Hepatic flexure
D) Splenic flexure

9.5. Which of the following organs is **not** part of the urinary (renal) system?

A) Kidneys
B) Bladder
C) Ureters
D) Liver

9.6. The estimated glomerular filtration rate (eGFR) is routinely used in clinical practice to assess renal function. This estimate of glomerular filtration rate (GFR) is calculated using which of the following variables?

A) Age and sex
B) Serum creatinine
C) Ethnicity
D) All of the above

Chronic kidney disease (CKD) can be classified into five stages, based on the level of renal function as measured by the estimated glomerular filtration rate (eGFR). These five stages can be seen in the following table:

Stage of CKD	GFR (ml/min/1.73m^2)
Stage 1	90+
Stage 2	60-89
Stage 3a	45-59
Stage 3b	30-44
Stage 4	15-29
Stage 5	< 15

9.7. If a patient has an eGFR of 27ml/min/1.73m², which stage of CKD would they have?

   A) Stage 3a
   B) Stage 3b
   C) Stage 4
   D) Stage 5

9.8. Which of the following signs or symptoms is a presenting feature of chronic kidney disease (CKD)?

   A) Bone pain
   B) Oedema
   C) Nocturia (excessive urination at night)
   D) All of the above

9.9. The clinical management of chronic kidney disease (CKD) involves multiple interventions geared towards reducing disease progression and correcting the metabolic complications of CKD. Sodium bicarbonate tablets would be given to treat which of the following complications of CKD?

   A) Anaemia
   B) Metabolic acidosis
   C) Metabolic bone disease
   D) Hyperkalaemia

9.10. Which of the following is **not** a function of the kidneys?

   A) Excretion of the end-products of metabolism
   B) Acid-base balance
   C) Albumin synthesis
   D) Bone metabolism

9.11. Resistance of the renal tubules to the action of antidiuretic hormone (ADH) is seen in which of the following disorders?

   A) Nephrogenic diabetes insipidus (nephrogenic DI)
   B) Type I diabetes mellitus
   C) Type II diabetes mellitus
   D) All of the above

9.12. Which of the following terms would be used to describe daily urine output in the range of 300-350ml?

A) Anuria
B) Oliguria
C) Polyuria
D) Normal urine output

9.13. It is important to assess the volume status of patients with renal disease, as this will determine whether fluids need to be given for routine maintenance, replacement or resuscitation. Following clinical examination, which of the following signs or symptoms would you expect to see in a patient with **hypervolemia**?

A) Prolonged capillary refill time (>2 seconds)
B) Increased weight
C) Reduced urine output
D) Hypotension

9.14. A number of different imaging modalities can be employed to detect and assess renal disease. Which of the following radiological investigations poses the **greatest** risk of nephrotoxicity?

A) Renal tract ultrasound when it is used to assess kidney size and identify cysts, tumours or obstructions in the urinary system
B) Abdominal x-ray when it is used to identify renal stones or calcification
C) A computed tomography (CT) scan with iodinated contrast, when it is used to investigate a patient with chronic kidney disease (CKD)
D) Magnetic resonance angiography (MRA) when it is used to look at the blood supply to the kidneys

9.15. The classic triad of oedema, hypoalbuminaemia (low plasma or serum albumin levels) and proteinuria (loss of protein in the urine) is seen in which of the following renal disorders?

A) Nephrotic syndrome
B) Nephritic syndrome
C) Pyelonephritis
D) Renal artery stenosis (RAS)

9.16. Which of the following is the most common cause of chronic kidney disease (CKD), leading to end stage kidney disease (ESKD)?

- A) Polycystic kidney disease (PKD)
- B) Renal vascular disease
- C) Diabetes mellitus (DM)
- D) Glomerular disease

9.17. Which of the following terms is used to describe a rapid, but often reversible, reduction in kidney function that occurs over hours to days?

- A) Acute kidney injury (AKI)
- B) Chronic kidney disease (CKD)
- C) Renal osteodystrophy
- D) Polycystic kidney disease (PKD)

9.18. Acute kidney injury (AKI) can be divided into three anatomic categories (pre-renal, intrinsic or renal and post-renal), based on aetiology. Which of the following is a **post-renal** cause of AKI?

- A) Glomerulonephritis
- B) Hypotension
- C) Kidney stones
- D) Hypovolemia

9.19. Kidney stones or renal calculi can be classified into four major types of stone: calcium, struvite, urate and cystine. Which of these crystalline stones is the most common?

- A) Calcium stones
- B) Struvite stones
- C) Cystine stones
- D) Urate stones

9.20. Hyperkalaemia is a common and potentially life-threatening metabolic complication of acute kidney injury (AKI). Which of the following statements is **true** with regard to this recognised complication of AKI?

- A) It can result in life-threatening arrhythmias
- B) The changes seen on an electrocardiogram (ECG) include tall, peaked and symmetrical ('tented') T waves, flattened P waves, widened QRS complexes and a prolonged PR interval
- C) A and B
- D) None of the above

9.21. Which of the following statements is **false** with regard to the actions of the proximal convoluted tubule and acid-base metabolism?

A) The reabsorption of filtered bicarbonate predominantly occurs in the proximal convoluted tubule
B) Carbonic anhydrase stimulates bicarbonate reabsorption
C) Acetazolamide is a carbonic anhydrase inhibitor with mild diuretic activity
D) An inability to reabsorb filtered bicarbonate can lead to metabolic alkalosis

9.22. Which of the following statements is **true** with regard to the urinary concentrating mechanisms in the kidney?

A) An osmotic gradient is generated and maintained in the renal medulla by the countercurrent mechanism
B) Urea accounts for up to 90% of the hyperosmolarity in medullary interstitial fluid
C) The kidneys concentrate urine during periods of increased fluid intake
D) Antidiuretic hormone (ADH) or vasopressin increases water reabsorption by decreasing the permeability of the collecting ducts

9.23. Which of the following statements is **false** with regard to the actions of the cortical collecting duct and the maintenance of fluid and electrolyte balance?

A) Sodium is reabsorbed in exchange for potassium in the cortical collecting duct
B) Aldosterone stimulates sodium reabsorption and potassium excretion
C) Spironolactone is an aldosterone antagonist and potassium sparing diuretic
D) Hypokalaemia is a predominant side effect of spironolactone use

9.24. There are numerous systemic manifestations associated with chronic kidney disease (CKD). Fatigue and pallor are associated with which of the following signs and symptoms of CKD?

A) Anaemia
B) Platelet abnormality
C) Hypertension
D) Infertility

CHAPTER 9

The Renal System (MCQs)

Answers and Detailed Solutions

The difficulty rating for each question (Easy, Moderate or Hard) can be found in parentheses next to the correct answer.

9.1. D (Moderate)

The kidneys are retroperitoneal structures located on the posterior abdominal wall, either side of the vertebral column between the last thoracic vertebra (T12) and the third lumbar vertebra (L3). The left kidney lies at a higher level than the right kidney, and healthy kidneys tend to be around 10-11cm in length. In addition, the kidneys are protected from trauma by the thoracic cage (rib cage).

9.2. B (Hard)

The glomerulus is a knot of capillaries located in the Bowman's capsule, within the renal cortex (not the renal medulla). The afferent (carrying towards) arteriole, a branch of the interlobular artery, enters the Bowman's capsule and branches into the glomerular capillaries. The distal end of the glomerular capillaries then reunite to form an efferent (carrying away) arteriole, which leaves the glomerulus. The renal tubule consists of several segments. Nearest to the glomerulus is the proximal tubule, followed by the loop of Henle and the distal convoluted tubule, which connects to the collecting duct system.

9.3. D (Hard)

The adrenal or suprarenal glands are highly vascularised. Along these lines, they receive blood from the inferior suprarenal arteries (inferior adrenal arteries), which branch off the left and right renal arteries, the superior suprarenal arteries (superior adrenal arteries), which branch off the inferior phrenic arteries, and the middle suprarenal arteries (middle adrenal arteries), which branch off the abdominal aorta.

9.4. C (Easy)

The spleen, stomach and splenic flexure of the colon lie in contact with the anterior surface of the left kidney. Conversely, the hepatic flexure of the colon, along with the liver and the duodenum, lies in contact with the anterior surface of the right kidney.

9.5. D (Easy)

The urinary (renal) system is composed of two kidneys and the urinary tract, which includes two ureters, the urinary bladder and the urethra. Accordingly, the liver is not part of the urinary system.

9.6. D (Easy)

The calculation of estimated glomerular filtration rate (eGFR) depends upon the patient's age, sex, ethnicity and serum creatinine. The value obtained correlates with the % of kidney function.

9.7. C (Easy)

Stage 1 chronic kidney disease (CKD) patients will have a glomerular filtration rate (GFR) of more than or the same as 90ml/min/1.73m². This indicates normal kidney function, although urine findings (such as protein in the urine) or structural abnormalities may point to renal disease. Stage 2 CKD patents will have a GFR of 60-89ml/min/1.73m². This indicates mildly reduced kidney function but other findings (similar to those seen in stage 1) may point to renal disease. Stage 3 is divided into 3a and 3b, with patients having a GFR of 45-59 and 30-44ml/min/1.73m² respectively. Stage 3a indicates a mild-moderate reduction in kidney function, while stage 3b indicates a moderate-severe reduction in kidney function. Stage 4 CKD patients will have a GFR of 15-29ml/min/1.73m². This indicates severely reduced kidney function. Stage 5 CKD patients will have a GFR of less than 15ml/min/1.73m². This indicates a very severe reduction in kidney function and end stage kidney disease (ESKD). Renal replacement therapy (RRT) is a necessity in these patients. Drawing these different threads together, it can be concluded that the patient in this question has stage 4 CKD and, as such, has severely reduced kidney function.

9.8. D (Easy)

Bone pain (metabolic bone disease), oedema and nocturia are all presenting features of chronic kidney disease (CKD). It is important to note, however, that chronic kidney disease is a silent disease and, as such, can remain asymptomatic or clinically silent in the early stages.

9.9. B (Moderate)

Metabolic acidosis is a common complication of chronic kidney disease (CKD). As CKD progresses, the kidneys gradually lose the ability to regenerate bicarbonate, creating an acid environment in the body, which impairs cellular function. Accordingly, sodium bicarbonate tablets can be given to help manage this acid-base imbalance. Vitamin D analogues, which increase calcium absorption, such as alfacalcidol, can be given to treat metabolic bone disease. Similarly, recombinant erythropoietin injections can be given to treat anaemia, along with iron (ferrous sulphate) tablets. In patients at risk of hyperkalaemia, it is advisable to reduce dietary intake of foods high in potassium (such as bananas and tomatoes).

9.10. C (Moderate)

The kidneys excrete the end-products of metabolism, such as creatinine, the end product of the catabolism of creatine, an amino acid found abundantly in muscle, and urea derived from amino acid breakdown. The kidneys also contribute to homeostasis by regulating acid-base balance through the alternation of hydrogen ion excretion and the reabsorption of bicarbonate. Moreover, the kidneys play a key role in bone metabolism, as naturally occurring vitamin D (cholecalciferol) requires hydroxylation, first in the liver and then the kidneys, to form 25-hydroxy cholecalciferol and 1,25-hydroxy cholecalciferol respectively. These two stages are important as the activated form of vitamin D (1,25-hydroxy cholecalciferol), which is secreted in the kidneys, is needed for the absorption of calcium from the gut. In contrast, albumin is synthesised in the liver (not the kidneys).

9.11. A (Moderate)

Nephrogenic diabetes insipidus (nephrogenic DI) is marked by resistance to the action of antidiuretic hormone (ADH) or vasopressin in the renal tubules, resulting in decreased water reabsorption in the kidneys. Accordingly, it is characterised by polyuria (a urine output that is greater than 3 litres per day, despite normal fluid intake) and polydipsia (excessive thirst). In addition, nephrogenic DI can be caused by drugs such as lithium.

9.12. B (Moderate)

A patient is considered to be anuric, when they produce little or no urine (<100ml/24hr, <4ml/hr or in some definitions, <50ml/24hr). Abnormally low urine output (<400ml/24hr) is known as oliguria. In healthy individuals urine volume is closely matched to water balance as regulated by antidiuretic hormone (ADH) or vasopressin, and is typically around 800-2000ml/24hr. A urine output that is greater than 3 litres per day (>3000ml/24hr), despite normal fluid intake, is defined as polyuria.

9.13. B (Hard)

A prolonged capillary refill time (>2 seconds), and reduced urine output are typically seen in hypovolemia. Likewise, hypotension (low blood pressure), with a postural drop is common in hypovolemia. The pulse rate will also be raised, in an attempt to increase cardiac output (CO). Similarly, skin turgor will be increased, and the jugular venous pressure (JVP) will not be visible. Conversely, increased weight is seen in hypervolemia, along with an elevated jugular venous pressure, and crackles on the lung fields.

9.14. C (Hard)

Renal tract ultrasound is a first-line investigation for the detection of urinary obstruction. This non-invasive test can also be used to assess kidney size and identify any cysts or tumours. Abdominal x-ray can be used to identify renal stones or calcification. Likewise, magnetic resonance angiography (MRA) can be used to assess the blood supply to the kidneys. A computed tomography (CT) scan with iodinated contrast, however, should be avoided in patients with chronic kidney disease (CKD) or who are acutely ill, as they are at risk of developing contrast induced acute kidney injury (AKI) or contrast-induced nephropathy.

9.15. A (Moderate)

The classic triad of oedema, hypoalbuminaemia (low plasma or serum albumin levels) and proteinuria (loss of protein in the urine, >3g/24hr) is seen in nephrotic syndrome, and is caused by damage to the glomerulus. Membranous nephropathy is the most common cause of nephrotic syndrome in adults, while minimal change disease is the most common cause in children. Nephritic syndrome, or acute nephritis, often presents with haematuria, proteinuria, oedema and hypertension, as well as acute renal failure. Pyelonephritis, or upper urinary tract infection, is characterised by fever, loin pain and other evidence of systemic infection (rigors, nausea, vomiting and diarrhoea), with or without the signs and symptoms of lower urinary tract infection (dysuria, urgency, urinary frequency, nocturia, haematuria, polyuria and supra-pubic pain). Renal artery stenosis (RAS) describes a narrowing of the lumen of one or both of the renal arteries, commonly due to atheroma or arterial dysplasia, leading to downstream ischaemic renal injury, and activation of the renin-angiotensin-aldosterone-system (RAAS), resulting in hypertension.

9.16. C (Easy)

Polycystic kidney disease (PKD), renal vascular disease and glomerular disease are all recognised causes of chronic kidney disease (CKD). Diabetes mellitus (DM), however, is the most common cause of chronic kidney disease, leading to end stage kidney disease (ESKD). This is marked by a number of clinical features, such as proteinuria and retinopathy. Furthermore, around one third of patients develop diabetic nephropathy. In renal vascular disease, the blood supply to the kidneys is compromised, leading to ischaemia. Glomerular disease is characterised by inflammation in the glomerulus, which can lead to protein and blood being excreted in the urine. Polycystic kidney disease is an autosomal dominant disorder, in which the kidneys are damaged by the development of multiple cysts, which replace normal renal parenchyma.

9.17. A (Easy)

Acute kidney injury (AKI) describes an acute process in which there is a rapid reduction in kidney function that occurs over hours to days, but is often reversible. Chronic kidney disease (CKD) refers to a chronic process in which there is a long-standing (present for over 3 months) and progressive reduction in kidney function. Unlike acute kidney injury, where recovery of kidney function is often possible, reversal and subsequent recovery is unlikely in chronic kidney disease. Renal osteodystrophy or bone disease is a common sign of chronic kidney disease. For further information about polycystic kidney disease (PKD) refer to the detailed solution for question 9.16. in this chapter.

9.18. C (Moderate)

Pre-renal causes of acute kidney injury (AKI) are often associated with the blood supply to the kidneys, and inadequate renal perfusion. Intrinsic or renal causes of AKI refer to structural damage inside the kidneys themselves. Moreover, post-renal causes of AKI are often due to obstruction of the renal tract, anywhere from the renal pelvis to the urethra. Hypotension and hypovolemia are pre-renal causes of AKI in which pump failure and a reduction in blood pressure result in inadequate perfusion to the kidneys. Glomerulonephritis is an intrinsic cause of AKI, along with tubular necrosis, as it will affect the kidney itself, while kidney stones, along with ureteric obstruction, are post-renal causes of AKI.

9.19. A (Moderate)

The vast majority (70-80%) of renal calculi are calcium stones. High levels of urinary calcium (hypercalciuria) is the most commonly identified cause of calcium stone formation. This is often due to high levels of calcium in the blood (hypercalcaemia), excessive absorption of calcium in the gastrointestinal tract or an inability to reabsorb tubular calcium. Struvite stones account for around 15% of renal calculi, and are composed of magnesium, ammonium and phosphate. These arise due to recurrent urease producing bacterial infections. Urate stones (5-10% of all kidney stones) develop when there is an excess of uric acid in the blood (hyperuricaemia) and high urinary concentrations of uric acid crystals. Accordingly, these urate stones are common in individuals with gout. Cystine stones are rare and occur in patients with the autosomal recessive transport disorder, cystinuria, in which the kidneys are unable to reabsorb the dibasic amino acids cystine, arginine, lysine, and ornithine.

9.20. C (Hard)

Hyperkalaemia (an abnormally high serum potassium level) is a potentially fatal metabolic complication of acute kidney injury (AKI) and, as such, can result in life-threatening arrhythmias if undetected or poorly treated. Patients with hyperkalaemia will first develop tall, peaked and symmetrical ('tented') T waves, and their electrocardiogram (ECG) will then display flattened P waves, widened QRS complexes and a prolonged PR interval.

For further information about the different components of an ECG refer to the detailed solution for question 7.17. in chapter 7 and for further practice with ECG interpretation refer to questions 21.1.-21.6. in chapter 21.

9.21. D (Hard)

The reabsorption of filtered bicarbonate predominantly occurs in the proximal convoluted tubule. This is stimulated by the enzyme carbonic anhydrase. Acetazolamide is a carbonic anhydrase inhibitor with mild diuretic activity and, as such, this potent agent can be used to inhibit bicarbonate reabsorption in the proximal convoluted tubule. An inability to reabsorb filtered bicarbonate, as would be precipitated by the use of this drug, can lead to metabolic acidosis (not metabolic alkalosis).

9.22. A (Hard)

The counter current mechanism is responsible for the concentration of urine in the kidneys. Along these lines, an osmotic gradient is generated and maintained in the renal medulla by the counter current mechanism. The absorption of urea is integral to this process, as urea accounts for up to 50% (not 90%) of the hyperosmolarity in medullary interstitial fluid. The kidneys will concentrate urine during periods of decreased (not increased) fluid intake (i.e. when dehydrated). To this end, antidiuretic hormone (ADH) or vasopressin increases water reabsorption by increasing (not decreasing) the permeability of the collecting ducts.

9.23. D (Hard)

Sodium, along with H_2O and Cl^-, is reabsorbed in exchange for potassium in the cortical collecting duct. This process of sodium reabsorption and potassium excretion is stimulated by the steroid hormone aldosterone. Spironolactone is an aldosterone antagonist and potassium sparing diuretic and, as such, prevents sodium retention in exchange for potassium. Accordingly, hyperkalaemia (not hypokalaemia) is a predominant side effect of spironolactone use.

9.24. A (Easy)

The kidneys are responsible for the production of erythropoietin. In chronic kidney disease (CKD), however, the synthesis of erythropoietin is impaired due to high levels of scarring and fibrosis in the kidneys. This can result in anaemia, which will present with a number of clinical features, such as fatigue, pallor, tachycardia and shortness of breath (SOB). As plasma urea levels rise in CKD, it can also interfere with platelet aggregation and leave individuals at risk of bleeding and bruising. Scarring in the kidneys can also affect the control and regulation of blood pressure, leading to hypertension. In addition, fertility often declines as you develop CKD.

CHAPTER 10
Haematology (MCQs)

10.1. The blood is a viscous fluid that is pumped around the body by the heart and the circulatory system, consisting of numerous specialised cells, suspended in a circulating liquid fraction known as plasma. Which of the following is the most abundant cellular component of the blood?

A) Platelets
B) Red Blood cells (RBCs) or erythrocytes
C) Monocytes
D) Basophils

10.2. All terminally differentiated blood cells are derived from a common progenitor cell in the bone marrow: the multipotential haematopoietic stem cell or hemocytoblast. Two major lineages emerge from this undifferentiated stem cell: myeloid and lymphoid progenitors. Which of the following cells is derived from the common **lymphoid** progenitor?

A) Red blood cells (RBCs) or erythrocytes
B) Macrophages
C) Natural Killer (NK) cells
D) Neutrophils

10.3. What percentage of the total blood volume is composed of liquid plasma?

A) 35%
B) 45%
C) 55%
D) 65%

10.4. Blood groups are a classification system based on the presence or absence of particular antigens on the red blood cell (RBC) membrane. The ABO blood group system is based upon carbohydrate antigens present on the surface of the RBC membrane. An individual with type __ blood is known as a 'universal donor'.

A) A
B) B
C) AB
D) O

10.5. Blood group compatibility is of great importance in transfusion medicine. If an incompatible blood group is transfused then acute haemolytic reaction can result. Which of the following signs and symptoms is **not** a clinical feature of ABO incompatibility?

- A) Renal failure
- B) Hypertension
- C) Haemolysis
- D) Haemoglobinuria

10.6. Which of the following terms **best** describes a condition in which the total number of circulating red blood cells (RBCs) or their oxygen-carrying capacity is inadequate to meet the body's physiological requirements?

- A) Anaemia
- B) Hypoxia
- C) Ischaemia
- D) Infarction

10.7. The body responds to anaemia with a number of established compensatory mechanisms, which help to maintain tissue oxygenation. Which of the following is **not** a mechanism of adaptation to anaemia?

- A) Increased erythropoiesis
- B) Increased cardiac output (CO)
- C) Increased oxygen extraction
- D) Decreased levels of 2,3-diphosphoglycerate (2,3-DPG)

10.8. Anaemia can be classified into three main types, based on morphology: microcytic, normocytic and macrocytic. Which of the following is a cause of **microcytic** anaemia?

- A) Iron deficiency
- B) Vitamin B_{12} deficiency
- C) Folate deficiency
- D) Liver disease

10.9. Which of the following is a cause of **normocytic** anaemia?

A) Thalassaemia
B) Lead poisoning
C) Acute blood loss or haemorrhage
D) Alcoholism

10.10. Which of the following terms is used to describe a significant rise in the number of circulating red blood cells (RBCs) or erythrocytes?

A) Monocytosis
B) Lymphopenia
C) Polycythaemia
D) Plasmacytosis

10.11. The following physiological changes take place in pregnancy **except**:

A) Physiological anaemia
B) Gestational thrombocytopenia
C) Increased fibrinolysis
D) Increased procoagulant factors

10.12. The haemostatic process can be divided into two phases: primary and secondary haemostasis. The former involves platelet activation and aggregation, while the latter involves the coagulation pathway. Which of the following statements is **true** with regard to the activation of these two haemostatic mechanisms?

A) Platelets are activated by multiple agonists, such as collagen, thromboxane A2 (TXA2), thrombin and adenosine diphosphate (ADP)
B) The extrinsic coagulation pathway is triggered by contact activation, as negatively charged surfaces activate coagulation factor XII (Hageman factor)
C) The intrinsic coagulation pathway is activated following vessel damage, as the glycoprotein, tissue factor (TF), is expressed on the surface of cells and binds to coagulation factor VII (proconvertin)
D) All of the above

10.13. Which of the following diagnostic tests is used to measure the **extrinsic** coagulation pathway?

A) Bleeding time (BT)
B) Prothrombin time (PT)
C) Activated partial thromboplastin time (APTT)
D) Thrombin clotting time (TCT)

10.14. If a patient presents with a prolonged activated partial thromboplastin time (APTT), then a mixing study can be performed. The clotting test is thus repeated with a 50:50 mix of the patient's blood and normal plasma. If there is significant correction and the test normalises, then the original abnormal coagulation test result was likely due to:

A) Deficiency
B) Inhibition
C) A and B
D) None of the above

10.15. Which of the following is **not** a vitamin K-dependent clotting factor?

A) Factor II (Prothrombin)
B) Factor V (Labile factor)
C) Factor VII (Proconvertin)
D) Factor X (Stuart-Prower factor)

10.16. In the event of a warfarin overdose, patients are at increased risk of:

A) Venous thromboembolism
B) Arterial thromboembolism
C) Hypercoagulation
D) Bleeding

10.17. A hereditary deficiency in coagulation factor VII (proconvertin) is associated with which of the following inheritance patterns?

A) Autosomal recessive
B) Autosomal dominant
C) X-linked recessive
D) X-linked dominant

10.18. Haemophilia A is an X-linked recessive disorder, marked by a deficiency in which of the following coagulation factors?

A) Factor VII (Proconvertin)
B) Factor VIII (Anti-haemophilic factor)
C) Factor IX (Christmas factor)
D) Factor X (Stuart-Prower factor)

10.19. Thrombophilias are abnormalities in the haemostatic mechanism, which predispose individuals to thrombosis. Which of the following thrombophilias is most likely to predispose an individual to **arterial** thrombosis?

A) Protein C (PC) deficiency
B) Protein S (PS) deficiency
C) Antiphospholipid syndrome (APC)
D) Factor V Leiden

10.20. Which of the following is a well-established risk factor for **arterial** thrombosis?

A) Immobilisation
B) Active cancer or cancer treatment
C) Diabetes mellitus (DM)
D) Oral contraceptive pill (OCP)

10.21. The oxygen binding proteins myoglobin (Mb) and haemoglobin (Hb) are involved in oxygen storage and transport respectively. Which of the following statements is **false** with regard to the differences between these two oxygen binding proteins?

A) Myoglobin binds to oxygen in a non-cooperative manner
B) Myoglobin's affinity for oxygen is not dependent on pH or carbon dioxide concentration, but it is regulated by 2,3-bisphosphoglycerate (2,3-BPG)
C) Haemoglobin binds to oxygen in a co-operative manner
D) Haemoglobin's affinity for oxygen is dependent on pH and carbon dioxide concentration, and it is regulated by 2,3-bisphosphoglycerate (2,3-BPG)

10.22. Which of the following physiological changes will cause the Hb-O_2 dissociation curve to be displaced to the **right**?

- A) Decrease in 2,3-bisphosphoglycerate (2,3-BPG)
- B) Increase in 2,3-bisphosphoglycerate (2,3-BPG)
- C) Temperature decrease
- D) Rise in pH

10.23. Which of the following oral anticoagulants is a direct **thrombin** inhibitor?

- A) Dabigatran
- B) Rivaroxaban
- C) Apixaban
- D) Edoxaban

10.24. The fibrinolytic system allows clots to be broken down *in vivo*. Which of the following proteins is the **end-product** of the fibrinolytic cascade?

- A) Plasminogen
- B) Plasmin
- C) Tissue plasminogen activator (tPA)
- D) Urokinase plasminogen activator (uPA)

CHAPTER 10

Haematology (MCQs)

Answers and Detailed Solutions

The difficulty rating for each question (Easy, Moderate or Hard) can be found in parentheses next to the correct answer.

10.1. B (Easy)

Red blood cells (RBCs) or erythrocytes are by far the most abundant blood cell, and are responsible for oxygen transport. Platelets are small anucleate blood cells, involved in the blood clotting system. Basophils are rarely seen in the bloodstream, as these granulocytes are a remnant of the primitive immune system. In addition, monocytes are phagocytic and antigen presenting cells.

10.2. C (Hard)

Natural Killer (NK) cells (large granular lymphocytes), along with T and B-lymphocytes, are derived from the common lymphoid progenitor. In contrast, red blood cells (RBCs) or erythrocytes, macrophages and neutrophils are derived from the common myeloid progenitor.

10.3. C (Easy)

The liquid fraction of the blood, plasma, accounts for around 55% of the total blood volume. Accordingly, blood cells or formed elements (such as red blood cells or erythrocytes, platelets and white blood cells) account for around 45% of the total blood volume.

10.4. D (Easy)

Individuals with blood group O are known as 'universal donors' as they have no A or B antigens on their red cell membrane and, as such, their blood can be given to a recipient of any blood type. An individual with blood group AB, which has no antibodies in the blood plasma, can receive blood donations of any type and is therefore called a 'universal recipient'.

10.5. B (Moderate)

Haemolysis occurs in cases of ABO incompatibility. If we transfuse an incompatible red blood cell unit, which contains ABO antigens against which the recipient has preformed antibodies, then the transfused units will be haemolysed intravascularly. As the red blood cells are lysing, there will be a large release of haemoglobin into the blood, which will eventually need to be filtered by the kidneys. To this end, the kidneys can become overworked as they try to filter and excrete excess haemoglobin, leading to renal failure. This filtration process will also result in the release of haemoglobin into urine (haemoglobinuria). In addition, blood pressure will drop (hypotension) and heart rate will increase in an attempt to compensate for this fall in blood pressure.

10.6. A (Moderate)

Anaemia describes a condition in which the total number of circulating red blood cells (RBCs) or their oxygen-carrying capacity is inadequate to meet the body's physiological requirements. Hypoxia is a state of reduced tissue oxygen availability, while ischaemia refers to a pathological reduction in blood flow to tissues. Tissue necrosis caused by ischaemia is known as infarction.

10.7. D (Moderate)

In chronic anaemia, the kidneys respond by increasing the production of erythropoietin and thus stimulating erythropoiesis (the production of mature red blood cells). Likewise, there is increased oxygen extraction due to an increase (not a decrease) in the levels of 2,3-diphosphoglycerate (2,3-DPG). Cardiac output (CO) also increases. If these adaptation mechanisms fail or are inadequate to maintain tissue oxygenation, then tissue will become hypoxic.

10.8. A (Moderate)

In microcytic or hypochromic anaemia, as seen in iron deficiency, the red blood cells are small and pale, and their mean cell volume (MCV) is < 80 femtoliters (fL) and their mean cell haemoglobin (MCH) is < 27 picograms (pg). In macrocytic anaemia, as seen in vitamin B_{12} and folate deficiency (megaloblastic macrocytic anaemia) and liver disease (non-megaloblastic macrocytic anaemia), the red blood cell volume is raised and the cells are larger (MCV > 95 fL). Megaloblastic anaemia is a descriptive term for a characteristic cell morphology caused by impaired DNA synthesis.

10.9. C (Moderate)

In normocytic or normochromic anaemia, as seen after acute blood loss or haemorrhage, the red cell volume is normal and there is a normal amount of haemoglobin per cell (MCV 80-95 fL and MCH 27+ pg). Thalassaemia and lead poisoning are both causes microcytic anaemia, while alcoholism is a potential cause of non-megaloblastic macrocytic anaemia.

10.10. C (Moderate)

A significant rise in the number of circulating red blood cells (RBCs) or erythrocytes is described as polycythaemia. Primary polycythaemia is a distinguishing feature of the chronic myeloproliferative disorder, polycythaemia vera (PV). Secondary polycythaemia is often seen in hypoxic conditions, such as chronic lung disease and right-to-left cardiopulmonary shunts. Lymphopenia refers to a decreased number of lymphocytes, as seen after a bone marrow transplant, as lymphocytes are some of the last cells to fully regenerate after a bone marrow transplant. An increased number of monocytes is known as monocytosis. This is seen in tuberculosis (TB). Likewise, a significant increase in the number of plasma cells is known as plasmacytosis. This can be benign in origin, for example in an infection, or have a malignant cause, for example in myeloma.

10.11. C (Hard)

Pregnancy is a pro-thrombotic state and, as such, is marked by an increase in the number of procoagulant factors (such as plasma fibrinogen and coagulation factor VII), and a decrease in fibrinolysis. Platelet count also falls, often after 20 weeks' gestation, with thrombocytopenia at its most prominent in late pregnancy. It is important to note, however, that there is often no pathological significance to this physiological change, for mother or foetus. Accordingly, the mother will usually make a full recovery postpartum. Physiological anaemia is also a common feature of pregnancy. This is because the plasma volume expands at a greater rate than the red cell volume, resulting in haemodilution, which peaks at around week 32.

10.12. A (Hard)

Primary haemostasis involves platelet activation and aggregation. Along these lines, when a blood vessel's integrity is breached and bleeding occurs, platelets are activated by multiple agonists, such as collagen, thromboxane A2 (TXA2), thrombin and adenosine diphosphate (ADP). Secondary haemostasis involves the coagulation pathway. Although this haemostatic mechanism functions as one pathway, it is classically divided into extrinsic and intrinsic pathways, which converge to form a common pathway. The intrinsic coagulation pathway is triggered by contact activation, as negatively charged surfaces activate coagulation factor XII (Hageman factor), while the extrinsic coagulation pathway is activated following vessel damage, as the glycoprotein, tissue factor (TF), is expressed on the surface of cells and binds to coagulation factor VII (proconvertin).

10.13. B (Hard)

Prothrombin time (PT) is used to evaluate the coagulation factors involved in the extrinsic and common pathway, while activated partial thromboplastin time (APTT) is used to measure the coagulation factors involved in the intrinsic and common pathway. Thrombin clotting time (TCT) is used to look at the ability of thrombin to convert fibrinogen to fibrin. Bleeding time (BT) is a test of abnormal platelet function. Accordingly, defects in primary haemostasis will give rise to a prolonged bleeding time.

10.14. A (Hard)

A mixing study is a useful test to perform after an abnormal result in the clotting screen, to decide if the result is due to a coagulation factor deficiency or the presence of an inhibitor. Along these lines, if a prolonged activated partial thromboplastin time (APTT) is due to a coagulation factor deficiency in the patient's blood, then it will be corrected and the test will normalise, following the addition of normal plasma. Conversely, if there is non-correction and the test remains abnormal then it is likely to be due to an inhibitor (usually an antibody). This is because if there is an inhibitor in the patient's plasma, it will still be present and active in the 50:50 mix.

10.15. B (Easy)

The vitamin K-dependent clotting factors are factors II, VII, IX and X and, as such, they all undergo vitamin K-dependant carboxylation. This post-translational modification, which converts glutamic acid (Glu) residues to gamma (γ)-carboxyglutamic acid (Gla), enables these vitamin K-dependant proteins to bind to the platelet surface via calcium.

10.16. D (Easy)

Warfarin acts an anticoagulant or blood thinner by inhibiting the enzyme vitamin K epoxide reductase (VKOR), which is needed to recycle vitamin K. This results in vitamin K deficiency, and a concomitant reduction in the activity of the vitamin K-dependant clotting factors. In the event of a warfarin overdose, patients are thus at an increased risk of bleeding.

10.17. A (Easy)

Hereditary deficiencies in coagulation factor VII (proconvertin) are inherited in an autosomal recessive manner. Similarly, hereditary deficiencies in coagulation factors I, II, V, X and XIII are inherited in an autosomal recessive manner. Von Willebrand disease (vWD) is the most common heritable bleeding disorder, and is inherited in an autosomal dominant manner.

10.18. B (Easy)

Haemophilia A is an X-linked recessive disorder marked by a deficiency in coagulation factor VIII (anti-haemophilic factor), an important co-factor for FIXa. Haemophilia B, or the Christmas disease, is an X-linked recessive disorder marked by a deficiency in coagulation factor IX (Christmas factor).

10.19. C (Hard)

The heritable thrombophilias predominately predispose individuals to venous thrombosis (such as deep vein thrombosis and pulmonary embolism). In contrast, the acquired thrombophilia, antiphospholipid syndrome (APS), in which auto-antibodies are directed against negatively charged phospholipids, is associated with both arterial and venous thrombosis. Factor V Leiden, or inherited activated protein C resistance, is the most common familial thrombophilia. Patients with this single point mutation in the factor V gene are at increased risk of venous thrombosis. This is because patients with this mutation are resistant to activated protein C cleavage, which inactivates coagulation factor Va. Protein C (PC) and protein S (PS) are natural inhibitors of coagulation. Activated protein C (aPC) proteolytically inactivates coagulation factors Va and VIIIa, while protein S is a cofactor for activated protein C. Accordingly, deficiency in the coagulation inhibitors, protein C and protein S, results in an increased risk of venous thrombosis.

10.20. C (Easy)

Immobilisation is a risk factor for venous thrombosis, as this can lead to venous stasis, particularly around the valves in the blood. Likewise, active cancer or cancer treatment is a risk factor for venous thrombosis, as it can lead to the expression of tissue factor (TF) on multiple cells, such as monocytes, resulting in a procoagulant response. The oral contraceptive pill (OCP) is also a risk factor for venous thrombosis, as hormonal changes can lead to shifts in the levels of certain clotting factors. In contrast, diabetes mellitus (DM) is a well-established risk factor for arterial thrombosis, as it is associated with an increased atherosclerotic burden, and can precipitate a prothrombotic state through the glycation of proteins, which will alter the coagulation cascade.

[Although the risk factors above apply mainly to arterial thrombosis and venous thrombosis respectively, it is important to note that a degree of overlap exists between the risk factors for venous and arterial thrombosis.]

10.21. B (Hard)

Myoglobin (Mb) is very well-designed as an oxygen storage protein, while haemoglobin (Hb) is equipped to pick up and deliver oxygen to different parts of the body. Haemoglobin binds to oxygen in a co-operative manner, so the binding of one oxygen molecule facilitates the uptake of subsequent molecules. This system can also be easily controlled as haemoglobin's affinity for oxygen is dependent on pH and carbon dioxide concentration, and it is regulated by 2,3-bisphosphoglycerate (2,3-BPG). Conversely, myoglobin binds to oxygen in a non-cooperative manner. The affinity of myoglobin for oxygen is not dependent on pH or carbon dioxide concentration, nor is it regulated by 2,3-bisphosphoglycerate (2,3-BPG), as befits its primary function as an oxygen store in tissues.

10.22. B (Moderate)

If you increase the level of carbon dioxide in the blood or increase lactic acid levels, it will lower pH (increase H$^+$) and cause a rightward shift. Accordingly, a rise in pH will cause the Hb-O$_2$ dissociation curve to be displaced to the left. At higher temperatures, the Hb-O$_2$ dissociation curve will be displaced to the right, and accordingly favour the unloading of oxygen to tissues. Similarly, an increase in 2,3-bisphosphoglycerate (2,3-BPG) will cause haemoglobin to give up oxygen more readily and, as such, lead to a rightward shift of the Hb-O$_2$ dissociation curve.

10.23. A (Hard)

Dabigatran is a direct thrombin inhibitor and, as such, its inhibitory activity is directed at the active site of thrombin (without the need to work through antithrombin). Rivaroxaban, apixaban and edoxaban exhibit direct anti-Xa activity and, as such, directly inhibit the active site of coagulation factor Xa (without the need to work through antithrombin). Notice that the direct thrombin inhibitor above ends in the suffix -tran, while the other three anti-Xa agents end in the suffix -xaban.

10.24. B (Moderate)

The proteolytic enzyme plasmin (or fibrinolysin) is the end-product of the fibrinolytic cascade, and is responsible for the lysis (break down) of fibrin clots. Plasminogen is converted to plasmin by the two serine proteases: tissue plasminogen activator (tPA) and urokinase plasminogen activator (uPA). These two enzymes (tPa and uPa) are used therapeutically as clot-busting drugs, particularly in the treatment of stroke.

CHAPTER 11
Endocrinology (MCQs)

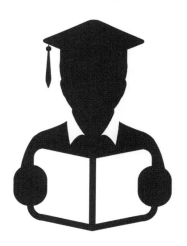

11.1. The anterior pituitary gland is under the control of the hypothalamus, and the secretion of hypothalamic releasing hormones, which have stimulatory or inhibitory action. Which of the following anterior pituitary hormones is under the **inhibitory** effect of the hypothalamus?

A) Growth hormone (GH)
B) Prolactin (PRL)
C) Thyroid-stimulating hormone (TSH)
D) Gonadotropins (FSH and LH)

11.2. Which of the following hormones is released by the **posterior** pituitary gland?

A) Antidiuretic hormone (ADH) or vasopressin
B) Oxytocin
C) A and B
D) None of the above

11.3. The adrenal glands are composed of two distinct types of endocrine tissue: the adrenal cortex (90% of the gland) and the adrenal medulla (10% of the gland). Which of the following hormones is produced by the adrenal **medulla**?

A) Catecholamines (adrenaline, noradrenaline and dopamine)
B) Mineralocorticoid (aldosterone)
C) Androgens (male hormones)
D) Corticosteroids (cortisol)

11.4. Which of the following signs and symptoms is **not** a clinical feature of adrenal failure (Addison's disease)?

A) Fatigue
B) Hyperglycaemia
C) Weight loss
D) Pigmentation

11.5. There are a number of distinctive clinical features associated with endogenous cortisol overproduction (Cushing's syndrome). Which of the following signs and symptoms are associated with the clinical presentation of cortisol **excess**?

A) Acne, abdominal striae, thin skin and easy bruising
B) Truncal obesity and extra fat deposits in the face (moon face), as well as around the neck and shoulders (buffalo hump)
C) Thin limbs, muscle weakness and growth arrest in children
D) All of the above

11.6. A number of different tests can be employed to investigate hormonal abnormalities. Stimulation tests can be used for suspected hormonal under-secretion and suppression tests can be used for suspected hormonal over-secretion. Which of the following is an example of a **stimulation** test?

A) A patient is given a steroid and their endogenous steroid production is subsequently measured
B) Adrenocorticotropic hormone (ACTH) is given to test for adrenal insufficiency
C) Dexamethasone is given for suspected cortisol overproduction
D) Glucose is given to test for growth hormone (GH) secretion

11.7. There are two biologically active forms of thyroid hormone: triiodothyronine (T_3) and thyroxine (T_4). Which of the following statements is **true** with regard to these two major forms of thyroid hormone?

A) Thyroxine (T_4) is the most biologically active form
B) Triiodothyronine (T_3) has little activity
C) Thyroxine (T_4) is deiodinated to triiodothyronine (T_3) in peripheral tissues by deiodinase enzymes
D) All of the above

11.8. Inappropriate stimulation of the thyroid gland by anti-TSH-autoantibody is seen in which of the following autoimmune diseases?

A) Graves' disease
B) Hashimoto's Thyroiditis
C) A and B
D) None of the above

CHAPTER 11: Endocrinology (MCQs)

11.9. Which of the following statements is **true** with regard to testicular hormone production?

A) Sertoli cells produce testosterone in response to luteinising hormone (LH) from the anterior pituitary gland
B) Leydig or interstitial cells produce inhibin in response to follicle stimulating hormone (FSH) from the anterior pituitary gland
C) A and B
D) None of the above

11.10. Hyperprolactinemia or prolactin over-secretion is a relatively common condition. It is often caused by a pituitary secreting tumour known as a prolactinoma. Which of the following is a clinical manifestation of prolactin **excess**?

A) Breast milk production (galactorrhea)
B) Menstrual disturbances in women (oligomenorrhea and amenorrhea)
C) Visual field defects
D) All of the above

11.11. Food intake and eating behaviour is controlled by hunger and satiety centres in the hypothalamus, and signals from orexigenic (appetite-inducing) and anorexigenic (appetite-suppressing) peptides. Which of the following hormones is an **orexigenic** agent?

A) Ghrelin
B) Leptin
C) Peptide YY (PPY)
D) Cholecystokinin (CCK)

11.12. In type I diabetes mellitus or insulin-dependant diabetes mellitus (IDDM), the primary defect is an inability to produce enough insulin due to the autoimmune destruction of pancreatic β cells. Which of the following is a characteristic of type 1 diabetes?

A) Late onset (commonly the 4th and 5th decades of life)
B) Gradual onset over many years
C) Strongly associated with being obese or overweight
D) Always requires exogenous insulin

11.13. In type 2 diabetes mellitus or non-insulin dependant diabetes mellitus (NIDDM), the primary defect is insulin resistance and β cell dysfunction. Which of the following is **not** part of the treatment plan for established type 2 diabetes?

A) Weight loss and exercise
B) Drugs that increase glucose secretion by the kidneys
C) Drugs that promote gluconeogenesis
D) Drugs that increase insulin sensitivity

11.14. The secretion of hormones in the hypothalamic-pituitary axis is regulated by multiple negative feedback loops. Which of the following statements is **false** with regard to negative feedback control and the modulation of hormone release?

A) High levels of circulating cortisol will switch off adrenocorticotropic hormone (ACTH) and corticotropin releasing hormone (CRH)
B) High levels of circulating thyroid hormones will switch off thyroid stimulating hormone (TSH) and thyrotropin releasing hormone (TRH)
C) High levels of circulating sex hormones will switch on follicle stimulating hormone (FSH), luteinising hormone (LH) and gonadotropin releasing hormone (GnRH)
D) High levels of circulating growth hormone (GH) will switch off growth hormone releasing hormone (GHRH)

The following **five** questions concern the effects of insulin and the counter-regulatory hormones on metabolism.

Insulin lowers blood glucose levels through a number of different mechanisms. There are, however, four major counter-regulatory hormones that act to increase blood glucose: glucagon, adrenaline, growth hormone (GH) and cortisol.

11.15. Which of the following statements is **true** with regard to the metabolic effects of the counter-regulatory hormones?

A) Adrenaline inhibits glycogenolysis
B) Adrenaline inhibits lipolysis
C) Glucagon stimulates glycogenolysis
D) Cortisol increases tissue glucose use

CHAPTER 11: Endocrinology (MCQs)

11.16. Glucagon increases blood glucose levels by stimulating:

A) Protein synthesis
B) Glycogen synthesis
C) Lipid synthesis
D) Gluconeogenesis

11.17. Glucose-stimulated insulin secretion leads to:

A) Glycolysis
B) Lipolysis
C) Proteolysis
D) Gluconeogenesis

11.18. Growth hormone (GH) stimulates each of the following metabolic processes, **except**:

A) Gluconeogenesis
B) Lipolysis
C) Proteolysis
D) Glycogen synthesis

11.19. An increase in circulating cortisol levels will promote:

A) Immunosuppression
B) Gluconeogenesis
C) Proteolysis
D) All of the above

11.20. Which of the following signs and symptoms is a presenting feature of hyperthyroidism?

A) Weight gain
B) Hand Tremor
C) Fatigue
D) Bradycardia

11.21. Which of the following signs and symptoms is a presenting feature of hypothyroidism?

A) Weight loss despite overeating
B) Tachycardia
C) Hyperhidrosis (increased sweating)
D) Constipation

11.22. Hypercalcaemia (an abnormally high level of calcium in the blood) is seen in which of the following disease states?

A) Acute Pancreatitis
B) Primary hyperparathyroidism (pHPT)
C) Secondary hyperparathyroidism (sHPT)
D) DiGeorge syndrome (22q11.2 deletion syndrome)

11.23. The renin-angiotensin system (RAS) or renin-angiotensin-aldosterone-system (RAAS) is a complex feedback system, which plays an important systemic role in the regulation of blood pressure, blood volume and electrolyte homeostasis. Activation of this system will result in:

A) Hypotension
B) Decreased sodium reabsorption
C) Increased aldosterone secretion
D) Decreased antidiuretic hormone (ADH) or vasopressin secretion

11.24. Which of the following is a clinical feature of Hashimoto's thyroiditis?

A) A smooth and symmetrical goitre
B) Unexplained weight gain
C) Exophthalmus (proptosis)
D) Heat intolerance

CHAPTER 11

Endocrinology (MCQs)

Answers and Detailed Solutions

The difficulty rating for each question (Easy, Moderate or Hard) can be found in parentheses next to the correct answer.

11.1. B (Hard)

Prolactin (PRL) does not have a stimulating hormone and is therefore under the inhibitory control of the hypothalamus. This lactogenic hormone is active after pregnancy, and stimulates breast milk production. The hypothalamus secretes thyrotropin releasing hormone (TRH), which tells the anterior pituitary gland to secrete thyroid stimulating hormone (TSH), which in turn stimulates the thyroid gland to produce thyroid hormones (triiodothyronine [T_3] and thyroxine [T_4]). Likewise, the hypothalamus secretes growth hormone releasing hormone (GHRH), which tells the anterior pituitary gland to release growth hormone (GH). Similarly, the hypothalamus secretes gonadotropin releasing hormone (GnRH), which tells the anterior pituitary gland to release follicle-stimulating hormone (FSH) and luteinising hormone (LH), which in turn stimulates sex hormone production by the testes and ovaries.

11.2. C (Moderate)

The posterior pituitary gland stores and releases two important hormones, which are produced in the hypothalamus. These posterior pituitary hormones are antidiuretic hormone (ADH) or vasopressin and oxytocin. Antidiuretic hormone stimulates the reabsorption of water by the kidneys when you are dehydrated, while oxytocin stimulates uterine contractions during childbirth, and the release of milk during lactation.

11.3. A (Hard)

The adrenal medulla comprises 10% of the adrenal gland and produces catecholamines (adrenaline, noradrenaline and dopamine). Conversely, the adrenal cortex comprises 90% of the adrenal gland and produces androgens (male hormones), corticosteroids (cortisol) and mineralocorticoid (aldosterone). The secretion of catecholamines (adrenaline, noradrenaline and dopamine) is not under the control of the pituitary gland, but connected to blood pressure. In like manner, the secretion of mineralocorticoid (aldosterone) is not controlled by the pituitary gland, but regulated by the renin-angiotensin-aldosterone-system (RAAS).

11.4. B (Moderate)

Adrenal failure (Addison's disease) is marked by an inability to produce sufficient levels of cortisol in response to stress. This is often due to adrenal atrophy and destruction, and is treated with long term steroid replacement. Individuals with adrenal failure are likely to exhibit a number of the following clinical features: fatigue, hypoglycaemia (not hyperglycaemia), weight loss, abdominal pain, constipation, pigmentation and hypovolaemic collapse. If undiagnosed, Addison's disease can prove fatal. Moreover, adrenal failure can be tested for by performing a stimulation test with synacthen, an adrenocorticotropic hormone (ACTH) analogue.

11.5. D (Moderate)

Skin abnormalities (acne, abdominal striae, thin skin and easy bruising), abnormal fat redistribution (truncal obesity and extra fat deposits in the face [moon face] and around the neck and shoulders [buffalo hump]), as well as thin limbs, muscle weakness and growth arrest in children are all part of the clinical presentation of Cushing's syndrome. Additional clinical features seen with cortisol excess include impotence and menstrual disturbances, glucose intolerance and psychiatric disorders (such as depression and psychosis).

11.6. B (Hard)

If you suspect that a patient has an under-active adrenal gland, this can be tested by stimulating the gland. If a large dose of adrenocorticotropic hormone (ACTH) is given and cortisol is subsequently measured, you would expect a rise in the cortisol level, if this does not happen then the patient is likely to have adrenal insufficiency. This is known as the synacthen test, and it is an example of a stimulation test. If you suspect growth hormone (GH) overproduction, then the glucose tolerance test can be used. If you give high levels of glucose to a patient, then growth hormone production should be inhibited. If you can still detect growth hormone, however, then hyper-function is indicated, as growth hormone production in a normal person would be undetectable. The glucose tolerance test is an example of a suppression test. Along similar lines, the dexamethasone suppression test can be employed to test for suspected cortisol overproduction, as seen in Cushing's syndrome. Dexamethasone is a strong steroid which, when administered, would be expected to suppress adrenocorticotropic hormone production in a normal individual. To this end, if the adrenal glands continue to produce cortisol after dexamethasone has been given, then cortisol overproduction is likely. Underlying this test is the principle that external steroids should switch off internal steroid production. Accordingly, if endogenous steroid production is measured and found to be high, after the administration of an exogenous steroid, then over-secretion is indicated.

11.7. C (Moderate)

There are two iodine-containing forms of thyroid hormone: triiodothyronine (T_3) and thyroxine (T_4). Thyroxine (T_4), which is metabolically inactive, is the major thyroid hormone in your circulation. This is deiodinated (converted) into the metabolically active form, triiodothyronine (T_3), in peripheral tissues by deiodinase enzymes.

11.8. A (Moderate)

Inappropriate stimulation of the thyroid gland by anti-TSH-autoantibody is seen in Graves' disease, and results in clinical hyperthyroidism. In contrast, Hashimoto's thyroiditis is an autoimmune process in which thyroid tissue is progressively destroyed, leading to hypothyroidism. In essence, antibodies stimulate the thyroid gland in Graves' disease, while antibodies destroy the thyroid gland in Hashimoto's thyroiditis, resulting in hyperthyroidism and hypothyroidism respectively.

11.9. D (Hard)

The testes are composed of Leydig or interstitial cells, Sertoli cells and seminiferous tubules, in which spermatogenesis takes place. Leydig or interstitial cells produce testosterone in response to luteinising hormone (LH) from the anterior pituitary gland. Conversely, Sertoli cells produce inhibin in response to follicle stimulating hormone (FSH) from the anterior pituitary gland.

11.10. D (Hard)

If you have a large pituitary tumour compressing the optic chiasma, then visual field defects often result. Likewise, breast milk production (galactorrhea) is seen in both men and women (90%). In addition, menstrual disturbances (oligomenorrhea) as well as the cessation of menstrual periods (amenorrhea) are seen in the majority of cases of prolactin excess.

11.11. A (Hard)

Food intake and eating behaviour is controlled by hunger and satiety centres in the hypothalamus, which are located in the lateral hypothalamic area and the ventromedial nucleus respectively. When the stomach is empty, ghrelin is released from neuroendocrine cells in the stomach to enhance hunger. In contrast, leptin is released from adipocytes to suppress hunger. Likewise, the gut hormones, peptide YY (PYY) and cholecystokinin (CCK) induce satiety and thus decrease food intake.

11.12. D (Easy)

Individuals with type 1 diabetes mellitus are insulin dependant and, as such, require lifelong exogenous insulin. Moreover, although type 1 diabetes can occur at any age, it typically has an early onset (around 10-14 years of age). This onset also tends to be rapid (days to weeks), and patients with the condition are usually slim. In contrast, type 2 diabetes mellitus is strongly associated with being obese or overweight, and has a late onset (commonly the 4th and 5th decades of life), which is gradual over a number of years. Most individuals will not need exogenous insulin, unless they have very severe type 2 diabetes.

11.13. C (Moderate)

Drugs such as metformin, which inhibit gluconeogenesis, are the mainstay of treatment for type 2 diabetes as they prevent the liver from over responding to the perceived lack of insulin. Drugs that increase glucose secretion by the kidneys and drugs that increase insulin sensitivity (such as pioglitazone), are also key oral anti-diabetic agents. The overarching aim of drug therapy is to reduce blood glucose levels. Weight loss and exercise are also crucial, and if substantial and consistent can actually reverse hyperglycaemia. If diabetes is poorly managed then individuals can experience a number of complications, such as retinopathy, chronic kidney disease (CKD) and coronary heart disease (CHD).

11.14. C (Moderate)

Negative feedback control is crucial to maintaining a constant internal environment (homeostasis). This regulatory mechanism detects deviations from the norm, and then triggers a response to counteract any changes and restore homeostasis. Along these lines, the examples in this question illustrate how negative feedback loops serve to keep hormone levels in balance. High levels of circulating thyroid hormones, for instance, will switch off thyroid stimulating hormone (TSH) and thyrotropin releasing hormone (TRH), so that the levels of thyroid hormone in the blood can return to normal. In like manner, high levels of circulating cortisol will switch off adrenocorticotropic hormone (ACTH) and corticotropin releasing hormone (CRH). Similarly, high levels of circulating sex hormones will switch off follicle stimulating hormone (FSH), luteinising hormone (LH) and gonadotropin releasing hormone (GnRH), and high levels of circulating growth hormone (GH) will switch off growth hormone releasing hormone (GHRH).

11.15. C (Easy)

Glucagon and adrenaline increase blood glucose levels by stimulating glycogenolysis and increasing lipolysis. In addition, cortisol raises blood glucose levels by reducing tissue glucose use.

11.16. D (Easy)

Glucagon drives the breakdown of glycogen, lipids and proteins in order to raise blood glucose levels. It also raises blood glucose levels via gluconeogenesis in the liver.

11.17. A (Easy)

Insulin is released in response to high blood glucose levels. In order to reduce blood glucose levels, it stimulates the synthesis of glycogen, proteins and lipids. Insulin thus inhibits gluconeogenesis, lipolysis, proteolysis, ketogenesis and glycogenolysis, and promotes glycolysis and cellular glucose uptake.

11.18. C (Easy)

Growth hormone (GH) stimulates lipolysis and gluconeogenesis. Furthermore, the hormone favours anabolism and, as such, promotes protein and glycogen synthesis.

11.19. D (Easy)

Cortisol is one of the major stress hormones, and is secreted by the adrenal gland whenever an individual is anxious or stressed. This hormone increases blood glucose levels by stimulating gluconeogenesis and proteolysis, and reducing tissue glucose use. Cortisol also has immunosuppressive effects.

11.20. B (Easy)

Hand tremor is a common symptom of hyperthyroidism. In contrast, weight gain, bradycardia (an abnormally slow heart rate) and fatigue are all associated with hypothyroidism, along with weakness and dry skin, hair loss and memory impairment.

11.21. D (Easy)

Weight loss despite overeating, tachycardia, hyperhidrosis (increased sweating) and heat intolerance are all associated with the clinical presentation of hyperthyroidism. Conversely, hypothyroidism is associated with weight gain, decreased sweating, the sensation of being cold and constipation.

11.22. B (Hard)

Primary hyperparathyroidism (pHPT), usually presents with high calcium levels (hypercalcaemia), with or without symptomatic renal and skeletal disease. In primary hyperparathyroidism, parathyroid hormone (PTH) reaches inappropriately high levels and this drives the reabsorption of calcium from urine by the kidneys, absorption of calcium in the intestines and the decomposition of bone, which releases calcium. Conversely, in secondary hyperparathyroidism (sHPT), the calcium level is usually either normal or low. This is a normal response to chronic hypocalcaemia, as the parathyroid gland tries to combat low blood calcium by boosting parathyroid hormone production via the process of negative feedback. If this process continues for a prolonged period of time, however, the parathyroid gland will eventually lose its ability to switch off, resulting in tertiary hyperparathyroidism (high blood calcium and inappropriately high parathyroid hormone). Secondary hyperparathyroidism is often caused by either chronic kidney disease (CKD), malabsorption or vitamin D deficiency. In addition, hypocalcaemia is a clinical feature of both acute pancreatitis and DiGeorge syndrome (22q11.2 deletion syndrome). The clinical presentation of hypercalcaemia is marked, albeit not exhaustively, by osmotic symptoms such as polyuria (passing too much urine) and polydipsia (excessive thirst), mood disturbance, constipation and abdominal pain.

11.23. C (Hard)

The renin-angiotensin system (RAS) or renin-angiotensin-aldosterone-system (RAAS) is stimulated by a fall in blood pressure, blood volume or blood sodium. When blood pressure drops, for instance due to blood loss following a road traffic accident (RTA), the juxtaglomerular apparatus in the kidneys sense this change and produce the enzyme renin. Renin then acts upon angiotensinogen, and converts this circulating substrate to angiotensin I (AI). Angiotensin-converting enzyme (ACE) is then released from the vascular endothelium in the lungs, and acts upon angiotensin I to form angiotensin II (AII). This octapeptide has several important functions. These include, arteriolar vasoconstriction and a subsequent increase in blood pressure, and the release of antidiuretic hormone (ADH) or vasopressin from the posterior pituitary gland, which will increase water retention in the kidneys. Furthermore, angiotensin II will stimulate the adrenal cortex to release aldosterone, which will act upon the kidneys to increase sodium reabsorption and water retention.

11.24. B (Moderate)

Hashimoto's thyroiditis involves the destruction of thyroid tissue by an autoimmune process, leading to hypothyroidism. It is common to gain weight when you have an under-active thyroid gland and, as such, individuals with Hashimoto's thyroiditis will often experience unexplained weight gain due to a fall in their metabolism. In contrast, the presence of a smooth and symmetrical goitre, heat intolerance and exophthalmus or proptosis (abnormal protrusion of the eyeball) are all associated with hyperthyroidism, and thus support a diagnosis of Graves' disease (not Hashimoto's thyroiditis).

CHAPTER 12
The Immune System (MCQs)

12.1. Which of the following constitutes the body's **first** line of defence against infection?

   A) Complement activation (the classical complement pathway, lectin complement pathway and alternative complement pathway)
   B) Antibody production
   C) Macrophages
   D) Physical barriers such as the skin and mucous membranes

12.2. Which of the following is an example of a **type II** (cytotoxic) antibody-mediated hypersensitivity reaction?

   A) Asthma
   B) Systemic lupus erythematous (SLE)
   C) Autoimmune haemolytic anaemia (AIHA)
   D) Contact dermatitis

12.3. Which of the following cells is **not** part of the innate immune system?

   A) Macrophages
   B) Natural killer (NK) cells
   C) Neutrophils
   D) Plasma cells

12.4. Which of the following is a major component of the **adaptive** immune system?

   A) Toll-like receptors (TLRs)
   B) C-type lectin receptors (CLRs)
   C) B cell receptors
   D) NOD-like receptors (NLRs)

12.5. The major lymphoid organs are functionally divided into primary (central) and secondary (peripheral) organs. Which of the following is a **secondary** lymphoid organ?

   A) Bone marrow
   B) Thymus
   C) Spleen
   D) None of the above

12.6. Monocytes are produced in the bone marrow, circulate in the bloodstream, and then migrate into surrounding tissues to mature into:

A) Kupffer cells (KC)
B) Macrophages
C) Langerhans cells (LC)
D) Microglia

12.7. Antibodies belong to a family of plasma proteins known as immunoglobulins (Igs). Which of the following is the **first** immunoglobulin class to be produced following infection?

A) IgA
B) IgD
C) IgG
D) IgM

12.8. Which of the following immunoglobulins (Igs) is able to cross the placenta?

A) IgG
B) IgA
C) IgD
D) IgM

12.9. Which of the following terms **best** describes a clinical situation in which the immune system is insufficient to protect the body against infection?

A) Immunomodulation
B) Immunodeficiency
C) Autoinflammation
D) Autoimmunity

12.10. Which of the following statements is **false** with regard to the differences between the innate and adaptive immune system?

A) Innate immunity is characterised by a fast response (hours to days)
B) Adaptive immunity is highly specific and targeted against a variety of pathogens
C) Adaptive immunity is characterised by a slow response (days to weeks after a primary exposure)
D) Innate immunity has a strong immunological memory

12.11. In parasitic infections there is likely to be a marked elevation in which of the following cells in the blood?

A) Neutrophils
B) Eosinophils
C) Lymphocytes
D) None of the above

12.12. Coeliac disease (gluten intolerance) is mediated by which of the following immunoglobulins?

A) IgA and IgG
B) IgA and IgE
C) IgD and IgE
D) IgE and IgG

12.13. Asthma is mediated by which of the following immunoglobulins?

A) IgA
B) IgD
C) IgE
D) IgM

12.14. Autoimmune diseases can be broadly divided into two categories: systemic and organ specific. Which of the following is a multi-system autoimmune disease (or a 'connective tissue disease')?

A) Systemic lupus erythematous (SLE)
B) Myasthenia gravis (MG)
C) Pernicious anaemia
D) Hashimoto's thyroiditis

12.15. The classical complement pathway involves an enzymatic cascade of proteins that interact to sequentially activate other proteins, via the process of limited proteolysis. The end result of complement activation is the formation of:

A) Antigen-antibody complex
B) Membrane-attack complex (MAC)
C) Complement factor C5b
D) Complement factor C1

12.16. Which of the following complement factors undergoes auto-activation in order to initiate the alternative complement pathway?

- A) C3
- B) C4
- C) C5
- D) C5b

12.17. Which of the following pathogens expresses mannose on their cell membrane or envelope, and will accordingly trigger the lectin complement pathway by binding to mannose-binding lectin (MBL)?

- A) *Candida albicans (C. albicans)*
- B) Human immunodeficiency virus (HIV)
- C) Influenza A
- D) All of the above

12.18. Anaphylatoxins are pro-inflammatory, cleavage by-products generated during complement activation. Which of the following molecules is **not** an anaphylatoxin?

- A) C3a
- B) C3b
- C) C4a
- D) C5a

12.19. Macrophages exists in three general states (resting, primed and hyperactive). Which of the following statements is **false** with regard to the contrasts between these different states of macrophage activation?

- A) The resting macrophage will take up larger objects by phagocytosis than the primed macrophage
- B) The primed macrophage expresses higher levels of major histocompatibility complex (MHC) class II molecule on its membrane than the resting macrophage
- C) Hyperactive macrophages are much larger than primed macrophages, and exhibit a higher rate of phagocytosis
- D) Hyperactive macrophages produce cytokines such as interleukin-1 (IL-1) and tumour necrosis factor (TNF), which kill both pathogens and tumour cells

12.20. Which of the following T cells express CD8 proteins on their surface, and are thus known as CD8+ T cells?

A) Cytotoxic or killer T cells
B) Helper T cells
C) Regulatory T cells
D) None of the above

12.21. Major histocompatibility complex (MHC) molecules, also known as human leucocyte antigens (HLAs), are a family of glycoproteins present on the surface of mammalian cells that help to differentiate self from non-self. These proteins play a critical role in T cell activation, as T cells will only see antigens in association with MHC proteins. Which of the following statements is **true** with regard to antigen presentation to T cells and MHC class?

A) Major histocompatibility complex (MHC) class I proteins present peptides to helper T cells
B) Major histocompatibility complex (MHC) class II proteins present peptides to cytotoxic or killer T cells
C) A and B
D) None of the above

12.22. The antigen-driven activation, proliferation and differentiation of naive B cells produces which of the following terminally differentiated cells?

A) Plasma cells
B) Memory cells
C) A and B
D) None of the above

12.23. Which of the following terms is used to describe antibodies that recognise and bind to multiple different epitopes (antibody-binding sites) on the same target molecule?

A) Monoclonal
B) Polyclonal
C) Paratopes
D) None of the above

12.24. Cytokines are a family of regulatory proteins involved in cell-cell communication. Which of the following statements is **false** with regard to these intercellular signalling molecules?

A) They are produced by T cells but not B cells
B) They activate B cells (leading to antibody production), T cells and macrophages
C) They function by drawing cells to a site of injury and then activating them
D) They exhibit pro-inflammatory and anti-inflammatory activity

CHAPTER 12

The Immune System (MCQs)

Answers and Detailed Solutions

The difficulty rating for each question (Easy, Moderate or Hard) can be found in parentheses next to the correct answer.

12.1. D (Easy)

Physical barriers such as the skin and mucous membranes constitute the body's first line of defence against infection. The innate immune system is the body's second line of defence. This includes the phagocytic activity of macrophages and complement activation (the classical complement pathway, lectin complement pathway and alternative complement pathway). Thereafter, the adaptive immune system provides a crucial line of defence against infection. Antibody (Ab) or immunoglobulin (Ig) production is an integral component of adaptive immunity.

12.2. C (Hard)

Autoimmune haemolytic anaemia (AIHA) is an example of a type II hypersensitivity reaction and, as such, is an antibody-mediated cytotoxic reaction. Contact dermatitis is an example of a type IV (delayed) T cell mediated hypersensitivity reaction, while asthma is an example of a type I immunoglobulin E (IgE) mediated hypersensitivity reaction. Likewise, systemic lupus erythematous (SLE) is an example of a type III immune complex mediated hypersensitivity reaction.

12.3. D (Easy)

Macrophages, neutrophils and natural killer (NK) cells are all part of the innate immune system. Macrophages reside in tissues, and are a first line of defence against pathogens. They engulf bacteria by phagocytosis, and release cytokines, such as tumour necrosis factor (TNF) and interleukin-1 (IL-1), once activated. Neutrophils normally reside in the bloodstream, and are summoned to the site of invasion and activated in response to signals from macrophages and bacteria, leading to the release of cytokines (such as TNF). Once activated (like macrophages) they will engulf bacteria by phagocytosis. Natural killer cells are another type of cell that are summoned from the blood. They also release cytokines, such as interferon gamma (IFN-γ) and interleukin-2 (IL-2), which will activate other cells. If a cell is infected by a virus then natural killer cells will trigger programmed cell death (apoptosis), in order to prevent viral replication and spread. In contrast, plasma cells are a type of B cell found in the adaptive immune system and involved in antibody production.

12.4. C (Easy)

Toll-like receptors (TLRs), C-type lectin receptors (CLRs) and NOD-like receptors (NLRs) are all pattern recognition receptors (or antigen recognition receptors). These pathogen recognition molecules are a major component of the innate immune system. Conversely, B cell receptors (BCRs) are a fundamental component of the adaptive immune system, and thus integral to the humoral (antibody-mediated) response.

12.5. C (Easy)

The sites of lymphocyte development and maturation are known as the primary (central) lymphoid organs. These include the thymus (in which T cells mature) and the bone marrow (in which B cells mature). Secondary (peripheral) lymphoid organs, such as the spleen, are associated with the immune response of mature lymphocytes.

12.6. B (Moderate)

Monocytes are produced in the bone marrow, circulate in the bloodstream, and then migrate into surrounding tissues to mature into macrophages. Macrophages then have different names in different tissues. They are known as Kupffer cells (KC) in the liver, Langerhans cells (LC) in the skin, microglia in the brain, osteoclasts in bone and alveolar macrophages in the lungs.

12.7. D (Moderate)

Immunoglobulin M (IgM) is the first immunoglobulin class to be produced following infection, and is thus associated with the acute setting of an infection. This initial antibody response typically appears within a week, and disappears after a few months. In contrast, immunoglobulin G (IgG) is indicative of past infection and long-term immunity. This delayed antibody response appears 10-14 days after infection and persists throughout life as part of an individual's immunological memory. Accordingly, if a patient has high levels of IgM and low levels of IgG for a specific antigen, then it will likely be due to a recent infection. Conversely, if a patient has high levels of IgG and low levels of IgM for a specific antigen, then it is likely to be due to an old infection or a response to vaccination.

12.8. A (Moderate)

Immunoglobulin G (IgG) is the only immunoglobulin that is able to cross the placenta and, as such, provides the neonate with naturally acquired immunity. Immunoglobulin A, D and M (IgA, IgD and IgM) are all found in breast milk and, as such, provide passive immunity to the newborn.

12.9. B (Easy)

Immunodeficiency describes a clinical situation in which the immune system is insufficient to protect the body against infection. Immunomodulation refers to the act of manipulating the immune system in order to achieve a desired immunological response, often through the use of immunity modulating agents. Autoimmunity and autoinflammation are associated with immunological disruption of the adaptive and innate immune system respectively. The former occurs when there is a break down in self-tolerance and the adaptive immune system inappropriately recognises and responds to the body's own cells and tissues, while the latter is characterised by seemingly unprovoked attacks of systemic inflammation.

12.10. D (Easy)

Adaptive or acquired immunity has a strong immunological memory, while innate immunity has no memory. For this reason, the adaptive immune system is able to mount a highly specific and targeted response against a variety of pathogens. In like manner, adaptive immunity is characterised by a slow response (days to weeks after a primary exposure) and innate immunity is characterised by a fast response (hours to days).

12.11. B (Moderate)

Marked elevations in eosinophil count (eosinophilia) are commonly seen in parasitic infections, such as schistosomiasis (bilharzia). Significant elevations in neutrophil count are often seen in bacterial infections, such as pneumococcal pneumonia, while an elevation in lymphocyte count is likely to be seen in viral infections, such as Epstein-Barr virus (EBV), which causes glandular fever or infectious mononucleosis (IM).

12.12. A (Hard)

Coeliac disease (coeliac sprue or gluten sensitive enteropathy) is an inflammatory condition induced by an autoimmune reaction to gluten. In contrast to the vast majority of food allergies, however, coeliac disease is not mediated by immunoglobulin E (IgE). Coeliac disease is mediated by immunoglobulins A and G (IgA and IgG) and, as such, can be diagnosed by testing for IgA or IgG antibodies to deamidated gliadin.

12.13. C (Easy)

Asthma is an immunoglobulin E (IgE) mediated, type 1 hypersensitivity reaction, characterised by inflammation and hyper-reactivity of the small airways. Accordingly, allergen-specific IgE tests can be employed as a diagnostic tool or to inform the treatment of asthma.

12.14. A (Easy)

Myasthenia gravis (MG), pernicious anaemia and Hashimoto's thyroiditis are all organ specific autoimmune diseases. Myasthenia gravis is an autoimmune disease in which autoantibodies are directed against acetylcholine receptors at the neuromuscular junction (NMJ). In pernicious anaemia, the absorption of vitamin B_{12} is impaired in the gut, as autoantibodies block the binding of vitamin B_{12} to intrinsic factor (IF). Systemic lupus erythematous (SLE) is a multi-system autoimmune disease (or a 'connective tissue disease') in which anti-nuclear antibodies form immune complexes in the circulation, which deposit in different organs, activating complement and causing inflammation. Hashimoto's thyroiditis is an autoimmune thyroid disease, in which thyroid follicles are destroyed leading to hypothyroidism. For further information about Hashimoto's thyroiditis (and Graves' disease) refer to the detailed solutions for questions 11.8. and 11.24. in chapter 11.

12.15. B (Moderate)

The classical complement pathway is activated by antigen-antibody complexes (which are generated by the adaptive immune system), and subsequently bind to complement factor C1. At the end of the classical complement pathway, complement factor C5b forms a complex with complement factors C6, C7, C8 and C9, forming the lytic membrane-attack complex (MAC). The MAC is a complex of several complement factors that perforate the cell membrane of pathogens or virus-infected host cells.

12.16. A (Hard)

The presence of bacteria will stimulate the auto-activation of complement factor C3, and subsequent release of C3b. Complement factor C3b binds to the bacterial membrane and the two proteins, factor B and properdin. This process then rapidly activities more C3 and C5, ultimately leading to the formation of a membrane-attack complex (MAC), in a manner akin to that seen in the classical complement pathway.

12.17. D (Hard)

The lectin complement pathway is activated by direct contact with pathogens that express the sugar mannose on their cell membrane or envelope, and subsequently bind to mannose-binding lectin (MBL). These pathogens include, albeit not exhaustively, the viruses (human immunodeficiency virus and influenza A), the yeast *(Candida albicans)* and bacteria such as *Salmonella*. Mannose-binding lectin then binds to MBL-associated serine protease 1 and 2 (MASP 1 & 2), which directly activate complement factors C2 and C4, ultimately leading to the formation of a membrane-attack complex (MAC), in a manner akin to that seen in the classical complement pathway.

12.18. B (Hard)

The anaphylatoxins (C3a, C4a and C5a) are cleavage-by products generated during complement activation. These pro-inflammatory molecules precipitate vasoconstriction through smooth muscle contraction, and trigger the degranulation of endothelial cells, mast cells (leading to the release of histamine) and phagocytes (which will release cytokines). C3a and C5a are also potent chemoattractants, which attract and activate neutrophils.

12.19. A (Hard)

Resting macrophages express low levels of major histocompatibility complex (MHC) class II molecule on their membrane. The primed macrophage thus expresses higher levels of major histocompatibility complex class II molecule on its membrane than the resting macrophage. This is important for antigen presentation. The primed macrophage takes up larger objects by phagocytosis than the resting macrophage and, in turn, hyperactive macrophages are much larger than primed macrophages, and exhibit a higher rate of phagocytosis. Hyperactive macrophages produce cytokines such as interleukin-1 (IL-1) and tumour necrosis factor (TNF), which can kill both pathogens and tumour cells.

12.20. A (Moderate)

Cytotoxic or killer T cells express CD8 proteins on their surface and are thus known as CD8+ T cells. Likewise, helper T cells express CD4 proteins on their surface and are known as CD4+ T cells. The role of regulatory T cells is not yet fully understood; it is believed, however, that they help to regulate and control the immune response in order to protect the body from self-destruction.

12.21. D (Moderate)

Major histocompatibility complex (MHC) class I proteins present peptides to cytotoxic or killer T cells, while major histocompatibility complex (MHC) class II proteins present peptides to helper T cells. Along these lines, antigens are processed and then presented together with MHC class I or II proteins to cytotoxic or killer T cells and helper T cells respectively.

12.22. C (Moderate)

The antigen-driven activation, proliferation and differentiation of naive B cells produces antibody secreting plasma cells and memory cells. The majority of B cells are transformed into plasma cells, which produce antibodies and secrete them into the circulation in order to fight infection. Memory cells remain in your bloodstream for a long time in case you encounter that particular antigen in the future and re-infection occurs, so that the immune system is ready to mount a quick and effective response.

12.23. B (Hard)

Polyclonal antibodies recognise and bind to multiple different epitopes (antibody-binding sites) on the same target molecule. In contrast, monoclonal antibodies will only recognise and bind to a single epitope on the same target molecule. Along these lines, polyclonal antibodies will target the same pathogen, but bind to different target sequences, while monoclonal antibodies possess the same target and the same target sequence. The antibody-active sites are known as paratopes or antigen-binding sites.

12.24. A (Hard)

Cytokines are a family of regulatory proteins, produced by B and T cells, albeit predominantly by the latter. Broadly speaking, these intercellular molecules function by drawing cells to a site of injury and then activating them. Accordingly, they activate B cells (leading to antibody production), T cells and macrophages. They also exhibit pro-inflammatory and anti-inflammatory activity.

CHAPTER 13
Microbiology and Infection (MCQs)

13.1. Which of the following statements is **true** with regard to the advantages and disadvantages of broad spectrum and narrow spectrum antibiotics?

A) There is a low risk of *Clostridium difficile (C. diff)* infection associated with the use of broad spectrum antibiotics
B) There is a high risk of *Clostridium difficile (C. diff)* infection associated with the use of narrow spectrum antibiotics
C) Narrow spectrum antibiotics can only be used to treat specific infections when diagnosis is either certain or there is strong clinical suspicion about the cause of infection
D) None of the above

13.2. Which of the following is the **first** stage of a typical viral life cycle?

A) Cell Entry
B) Attachment
C) Uncoating
D) Genome replication

13.3. Which of the following statements is **false** with regard to the structural and reproductive elements of fungal pathogens and the infections they typically cause?

A) Fungi are simple eukaryotic organisms, which reproduce via sexual or asexual sporulation (spore formation)
B) Most fungi possess a cell wall composed of cellulose and other polymers
C) Candida are a large genus of yeasts, implicated in the causation of superficial mucosal disease, as well as systemic disease
D) Dermatophytes are a group of keratinophilic fungi implicated in the causation of a great number of skin, hair and nail diseases

13.4. Rank the following organisms in order of size, from smallest to largest:

A) Protozoa, Bacteria, Prions, Helminths, Fungi, Viruses
B) Prions, Viruses, Bacteria, Fungi, Protozoa, Helminths
C) Fungi, Bacteria, Helminths, Viruses, Protozoa, Prions
D) Bacteria, Viruses, Protozoa, Fungi, Prions, Helminths

13.5. Helminths (worms) can be divided into three main classes: cestodes (tapeworms), trematodes (flukes) and nematodes (roundworms). Which of the following types of parasitic worm are segmented and flat?

A) Cestodes
B) Trematodes
C) Nematodes
D) None of the above

13.6. Parasites can be broadly classified into two types: ectoparasites and endoparasites. Endoparasites live inside the body of their host, while ectoparasites live outside or on the body of their host. Which of the following organisms is an **endoparasite**?

A) Lice
B) Fleas
C) Ticks
D) Protozoa

13.7. Viruses are obligate intracellular parasites and, as such, are totally dependent on their host cells for growth, survival and replication. Each virus consists of which of the following structural components?

A) An envelope (lipid bilayer) and protein coat (capsid)
B) A genome (DNA or RNA) and protein coat (capsid)
C) An envelope (lipid bilayer) and genome (DNA or RNA)
D) A protein coat (capsid) and viral enzymes

13.8. Malaria is a febrile, mosquito-borne illness caused by four species of the genus *Plasmodium*. Which of the following protozoan parasites is the most clinically severe?

A) *Plasmodium falciparum (P. falciparum)*
B) *Plasmodium vivax (P. vivax)*
C) *Plasmodium ovale (P. ovale)*
D) *Plasmodium malariae (P. malariae)*

13.9. Which of the following respiratory viruses is the most frequent cause of the 'common cold'?

A) Influenza viruses
B) Coronaviruses
C) Respiratory syncytial virus (RSV)
D) Rhinoviruses

13.10. Five primary hepatotropic viruses have been discovered to date: Hepatitis A, B, C, D and E. Which of the following is **not** a mode of hepatitis B transmission?

A) Sexual
B) Vertical
C) Faeco-oral
D) Parenteral

13.11. Cystitis (bladder infection) is a lower urinary tract infection (LUTI) commonly caused by infection with gut bacteria. Which of the following organisms is the most common cause of cystitis?

A) *Escherichia coli (E. coli)*
B) *Proteus mirabilis (P. mirabilis)*
C) *Staphylococcus saprophyticus (S. saprophyticus)*
D) *Pseudomonas aeruginosa (P. aeruginosa)*

13.12. Which of the following is a gram-positive bacillus implicated in the causation of antibiotic-associated diarrhoea?

A) *Staphylococcus aureus (S. aureus)*
B) *Clostridium difficile (C. diff)*
C) *Streptococcus pyogenes (S. pyogenes)*
D) *Treponema pallidum (T. pallidum)*

13.13. Which of the following is a double-stranded DNA virus implicated in the causation of chicken pox?

A) Herpes simplex virus 1 (HSV-1)
B) Herpes simplex virus 2 (HSV-2)
C) Human parvovirus B19 (B19V)
D) Varicella zoster virus (VZV)

13.14. Which of the following is a gram-negative spiral shaped bacterium implicated in the causation of gastritis and peptic ulcer disease (PUD)?

A) *Bordetella pertussis (B. pertussis)*
B) *Helicobacter pylori (H. pylori)*
C) *Borrelia burgdorferi (B. burgdorferi)*
D) *Streptococcus agalactiae (S. agalactiae)*

13.15. Symbiosis refers to a situation in which two or more organisms co-exist in close physical association. Which of the following terms **best** describes a symbiotic relationship in which one organism benefits but the other organism derives neither benefit nor harm from the association?

   A) Parasitism
   B) Commensalism
   C) Mutualism
   D) Neutralism

13.16. The body can be divided into sterile (contain no normal flora) and non-sterile (contain normal flora) sites. Which of the following is a **sterile** body site?

   A) Skin
   B) Vagina
   C) Urinary tract
   D) Nasopharynx

13.17. Which of the following terms is used to describe the ability of a microorganism to become established on or in a host?

   A) Infectivity
   B) Virulence or pathogenicity
   C) A and B
   D) None of the above

13.18. Which of the following statements is **false** with regard to the differences between endotoxins and exotoxins?

   A) Endotoxins are produced by living bacteria, while exotoxins are released from damaged or dead cells
   B) Endotoxins are a component of the outer membrane of gram-negative bacteria
   C) Lipopolysaccharides (LPS) are the most significant biologically active component of bacterial endotoxins
   D) Botulism and tetanus are examples of exotoxin-mediated diseases

13.19. Bacteria can be classified into two groups, based on whether or not their cell walls retain crystal violet when stained and washed with acetone. This is known as a gram stain, and it utilises the fact that bacterial cell walls vary in composition. If a bacterium is identified as gram-positive then which of the following statements would be **true**?

A) The gram stain is purple, as the purple stain is trapped inside the cell
B) The gram stain is pink, as the purple stain is not retained
C) The cell wall contains very little peptidoglycan (1-3 layers) and an extra, thick outer membrane
D) None of the above

13.20. Which of the following bacterial species is poorly visible using conventional gram staining?

A) Mycobacterium
B) Bacillus
C) Neisseria
D) Clostridium

13.21. Which of the following statements is **false** with regard to the basic structure of a bacterium?

A) They are unicellular, microscopic organisms, with a simple cell structure
B) Bacterial cells lack a membrane bound nucleus, and are known as eukaryotes
C) Motile bacteria contain organs of locomotion called flagella
D) Some bacteria are surrounded by a capsule or slime layer, which provides protection and facilitates adhesion to particular surfaces

13.22. The cell wall is a common target for antibacterial and antifungal agents. Which of the following statements is **false** with regard to the bacterial and fungal cell wall and the action of cell wall synthesis inhibitors?

A) Peptidoglycan is a major component of the bacterial cell wall and β-1,3-glucan is a major component of the fungal cell wall
B) β-lactam antibiotics (antibacterial agents), such as the penicillins, work by impairing the function of 'penicillin-binding proteins' (PBPs) - transpeptidase enzymes involved in the synthesis and maintenance of the peptidoglycan portion of the bacterial cell wall
C) Echinocandins (antifungal agents) work by inhibiting β-1,3-glucan synthase (the main enzyme used in the generation of β-1,3-glucan)
D) There is no cell wall in animal cells, so antibacterial and antifungal cell wall synthesis inhibitors are unable to demonstrate selective toxicity

13.23. Which of the following statements is **true** with regard to human immunodeficiency virus (HIV)?

A) The virus is present in the blood, genital secretions and breast milk of infected individuals, and can be transmitted sexually, vertically (from mother to child) and via needle stick injury
B) The virus targets helper T cells (CD4+ T cells)
C) It is a retrovirus as the enzyme reverse transcriptase (RT) converts its RNA genome into DNA, which can then be integrated into the host cell's genome by a viral integrase enzyme
D) All of the above

13.24. Human papillomaviruses (HPVs) are double-stranded DNA viruses capable of inducing benign genital warts, cervical carcinoma, anogenital cancers and some head and neck cancers. Genital HPVs can be divided into high and low risk groups, based upon their oncogenic potential. Which of the following are **high** risk HPV sub-types associated with cervical cancer?

A) HPV-6 and 11
B) HPV-11 and 16
C) HPV-16 and 18
D) HPV-11 and 18

CHAPTER 13

Microbiology and Infection (MCQs)

Answers and Detailed Solutions

The difficulty rating for each question (Easy, Moderate or Hard) can be found in parentheses next to the correct answer.

13.1. C (Easy)

Narrow spectrum antibiotics can only be used to treat specific infections when diagnosis is either certain or there is a strong clinical suspicion about the cause of infection. Accordingly, there is a low risk of *Clostridium difficile (C. diff)* infection associated with the use of narrow spectrum antibiotics. Broad spectrum antibiotics can be used to simultaneously treat more than one infection and are thus associated with a high risk of *C. diff* infection. This is because broad spectrum antibiotics (such as vancomycin) kill more normal flora than narrow spectrum antibiotics (such as nitrofurantoin and trimethoprim).

13.2. B (Moderate)

In broad brush strokes, a typical virus life cycle will be composed of the following stages. The virus attaches to the host cell (via a receptor), and cell entry occurs. Once the virus is inside the cell, it can be uncoated. The protein coat (capsid) will thus break down, and the genome will be released and targeted to the nucleus of the cell. Early viral proteins (such as viral enzymes) will then be produced. This is followed by genome replication, with viral genetic material being replicated in the host nucleus. Following this late stage viral proteins (structural proteins) will be produced. Virus assembly will then take place followed by virus release and maturation. Antiviral drugs work by blocking different stages of the viral life cycle.

13.3. B (Moderate)

Fungi are simple eukaryotic organisms, which reproduce via sexual or asexual sporulation (spore formation). In addition, the vast majority possess a cell wall composed of chitin (not cellulose) and other polymers. Cellulose is a major component of the plant cell wall, by and large absent from fungal cell walls. Candida are a large genus of yeasts, implicated in the causation of superficial mucosal disease, as well as systemic disease. Dermatophytes are a group of keratinophilic fungi implicated in the causation of a great number of skin, hair and nail diseases. These include, albeit not exhaustively, athlete's foot (tinea pedis), scalp ringworm (tinea capitis) and fungal nail disease (tinea unguium).

13.4. B (Easy)

In order of size from smallest to largest, the given organisms would be classified as follows: Prions, Viruses, Bacteria, Fungi, Protozoa and Helminths. Microscopy is required to view the majority of the organisms in the first half of this list, although organisms such as helminths (worms) are large enough to be seen with the naked eye. Viruses, for instance, can only be seen using electron microscopy.

13.5. A (Moderate)

Helminths (worms) can be divided into different groups based on their size and shape. Cestodes (tapeworms), such as *Taenia saginata* (beef tapeworm) and *Taenia solium* (pork tapeworm), are segmented and flat. Trematodes (flukes), such as *Schistosoma haematobium (S. haematobium)*, are unsegmented and flat. Nematodes (roundworms) are cylindrical and contain a simple digestive tract that runs from mouth to anus.

13.6. D (Easy)

Endoparasites, such as protozoa, live inside the body of their host and are a major cause of infection. In contrast, lice, fleas and ticks are ectoparasites and, as such, live outside or on the body of their host.

13.7. B (Moderate)

All viruses contain a genome or nucleic acid core (DNA or RNA), surrounded by a protein coat (capsid). Some, but not all, viruses have an envelope (lipid bilayer), while others are naked (non-enveloped) and have their protein coat exposed. In addition, some viruses contain their own enzymes.

13.8. A (Hard)

Malaria is a mosquito-borne, febrile illness, mainly present in tropical regions. Severe cases of malaria are, in the main, attributed to *Plasmodium falciparum (P. falciparum)*. If this form of malaria is suspected, then it should be considered as a medical emergency, as this micro-parasite can cause death and severe organ failure. The potentially fatal complications of infection with *P. falciparum* include, albeit not exhaustively, renal failure (black water fever), cerebral malaria (headache and confusion eventually leading to coma), severe anaemia, pulmonary oedema and circulatory collapse.

13.9. D (Easy)

Rhinoviruses (from the Greek 'rhinos', which means nose) are the most frequent cause of the 'common cold' (around 40% of cases). Respiratory syncytial virus (RSV) commonly affects young children, and is the leading cause of bronchiolitis in children under 2 years of age. This is an inflammation of the bronchioles, characterised by a cough, nasal discharge, wheeze, hypoxia and fever. Respiratory syncytial virus is implicated in around 5% of cases of the 'common cold'. Influenza (flu) viruses are responsible for roughly 10% of cases, while coronaviruses cause approximately 10-15% of cases.

13.10. C (Moderate)

Hepatitis A and E are transmitted by the faeco-oral route, as the viruses are shed in the faeces of infected individuals. These hepatotropic viruses tend to be self-limiting and resolve independently. Conversely, hepatitis B is a blood-borne virus, which can be spread via vertical (from mother to child), sexual or parenteral transmission. In contrast to hepatitis A and E, infection with hepatitis B (and hepatitis C) can progress to chronic hepatitis. If untreated, this can cause cirrhosis and eventually result in hepatocellular carcinoma (HCC).

13.11. A (Moderate)

The gram-negative bacillus *Escherichia coli (E. coli)* is the causative agent in most cases of cystitis (bladder infection). Infection of the lower urinary tract is marked by the following clinical features: urgency, frequency, dysuria or painful urination and lower abdominal pain.

13.12. B (Hard)

Clostridium difficile (C. diff) is a gram-positive bacillus implicated in the causation of antibiotic-associated diarrhoea (as well as antibiotic-associated colitis and pseudomembranous colitis). *Staphylococcus aureus (S. aureus)* is a gram-positive coccus, predominately found in the nose, which causes skin and soft tissue infections. *Streptococcus pyogenes (S. pyogenes)* or group A *Streptococcus* (GAS) is a gram-positive bacterium. It is also the most common cause of a bacterial sore throat, and a causative agent of scarlet fever. *Treponema pallidum (T. pallidum)* is a spiral bacterium which causes syphilis.

13.13. D (Hard)

Varicella zoster virus (VZV) is a double-stranded DNA virus and a member of the herpes virus family. Primary infection with varicella zoster virus is implicated in the causation of chicken pox, and 'herpes zoster' or 'shingles' if the virus is reactivated in later life. Herpes simplex virus types 1 and 2 (HSV-1 and HSV-2) are double-stranded DNA viruses associated with the development of cold sores and genital herpes respectively. Human parvovirus B19 (B19V) is a single-stranded DNA virus, and the causative agent of erythema infectiosum (fifth disease or slapped cheek syndrome), as well as transient aplastic crisis (TAC) in individuals with chronic haemolytic anaemia.

13.14. B (Hard)

Helicobacter pylori (H. pylori) is a gram-negative spiral shaped bacterium implicated in the causation of gastritis and peptic ulcer disease (PUD). It also has a strong association with gastric cancer. Bacterial infection with *H. pylori* is treated with a course of triple therapy. This consists of a proton pump inhibitor (gastric acid secretion blocker), such as omeprazole, combined with two antibiotics, such as clarithromycin and metronidazole. *Bordetella pertussis (B. pertussis)*, a gram-negative cocco-bacillus, is the causative agent of pertussis or whooping cough, a highly contagious disease that infects the respiratory tract. *Borrelia burgdorferi (B. burgdorferi)* is a spiral-shaped bacterium associated with Lyme disease. *Streptococcus agalactiae (S. agalactiae)* or group B *Streptococcus* (GBS) is a gram-positive coccus arranged in chains, and the most common cause of bacterial meningitis and sepsis in neonates.

13.15. B (Easy)

Commensalism describes a symbiotic relationship in which one organism benefits but the other organism derives neither benefit nor harm from the association. Parasitism refers to a situation in which one organism (the parasite) benefits at the expense of the other organism (the host). Mutualism describes a symbiotic relationship in which both organisms benefit from the association. By the same token, neutralism refers to a situation in which neither organism derives benefit nor harm.

13.16. C (Easy)

The skin, vagina and nasopharynx are all non-sterile sites as they are exposed to the environment (either directly or indirectly) and have no established mechanism in place to maintain sterility. In contrast, the urinary tract is a sterile site, as it is protected by the urethra, which helps to maintain sterility.

13.17. A (Easy)

Infectivity describes the ability of a microorganism to become established on or in a host. Virulence and pathogenicity may be used interchangeably to refer to the capacity of a micro-organism to cause an infection.

13.18. A (Hard)

Exotoxins are proteins produced by living bacteria, while endotoxins are released from damaged or dead cells. Along these lines, endotoxins are a component of the outer membrane of gram-negative bacteria, and lipopolysaccharides (LPS) are the most significant biologically active component of bacterial endotoxins. Botulism and tetanus are examples of exotoxin-mediated diseases. Botulism is caused by *Clostridium botulinum (C. botulinum)*, and can be precipitated by the ingestion of food contaminated with the toxin or the infection of a dirty wound. This exotoxin-mediated disease is marked by muscle weakness, and can present with diplopia, dysphagia, dysarthria and dry mouth. Equally, it can be fatal due to flaccid paralysis of the muscles of respiration. Tetanus is caused by *Clostridium tetani (C. tetani)*, and like botulism, is associated with the infection of dirty wounds. In contrast to botulism, tetanus causes a rigid paralysis (rather than a flaccid paralysis), which can be fatal if respiratory paralysis occurs.

13.19. A (Moderate)

If a bacterium is identified as gram-positive then the gram stain will be purple, as purple stain will be trapped inside the cell. Conversely, if a bacterium is identified as gram-negative then the gram stain will be pink, as purple stain will not be retained by the cell. These results can be explained by fundamental structural and chemical differences in the cell wall of a gram-positive and gram-negative bacterium. The cell wall of a gram-positive bacterium is very thick and consists of 30-40 layers of peptidoglycan, while the cell wall of a gram-negative bacterium contains very little peptidoglycan (1-3 layers) and an extra, thick outer membrane. The gram stain is of great clinical importance as it can help to guide which antibiotics are prescribed.

13.20. A (Hard)

Mycobacterium species, such as *Mycobacterium tuberculosis (M. tuberculosis)*, are poorly visible using conventional gram staining, as their lipid-rich cell wall resists uptake of the chemical dyes used in gram stain. Accordingly, Mycobacterium are often detected using the Ziehl-Neelsen (ZN) staining technique. Bacillus, Neisseria and Clostridium species can all be detected using conventional gram staining.

13.21. B (Easy)

Bacteria are unicellular, microscopic organisms, with a simple cell structure. Bacterial cells lack a membrane bound nucleus, and are thus known as prokaryotes (derived from Greek roots meaning 'before nucleus'), not eukaryotes (derived from Greek roots meaning 'true nucleus'). Motile bacteria contain organs of locomotion called flagella, and some bacteria are surrounded by a capsule or slime layer, which provides protection and facilitates adhesion to particular surfaces.

13.22. D (Hard)

There is no cell wall in animal cells, so antibacterial and antifungal cell wall synthesis inhibitors demonstrate selective toxicity (i.e. the target of the antimicrobial agent is not present or accessible in the human host). Peptidoglycan is a major component of the bacterial cell wall and β-1,3-glucan is a major component of the fungal cell wall. Along these lines, β-lactam antibiotics (antibacterial agents), such as the penicillins, work by impairing the function of 'penicillin-binding proteins' (PBPs) - transpeptidase enzymes involved in the synthesis and maintenance of the peptidoglycan portion of the bacterial cell wall. In like manner, echinocandins (antifungal agents) work by inhibiting β-1,3-glucan synthase (the main enzyme used in the generation of β-1,3-glucan).

13.23. D (Moderate)

Human immunodeficiency virus (HIV) is an enveloped retrovirus present in the blood, genital secretions and breast milk of infected individuals. The virus targets helper T cells (CD4+ T cells) and can be transmitted sexually, vertically (from mother to child) and via needle stick injury. It is known as a retrovirus because the enzyme reverse transcriptase (RT) converts its RNA genome into DNA, which can then be integrated into the host cell's genome by a viral integrase enzyme.

13.24. C (Hard)

HPV-16 and 18 are high risk viral subtypes responsible for approximately 70% of cervical cancers. In contrast, HPV-6 and 11 are low risk viral subtypes associated with benign genital warts and numerous other low grade cytological abnormalities. These HPV subtypes are the most clinically significant and, as such, HPV vaccines will often be specifically targeted against HPV-6, 11, 16 and 18.

CHAPTER 14
The Musculoskeletal System (MCQs)

14.1. The skeletal system is composed of highly specialised connective tissues, which perform a number of essential functions in the body. Which of the following is an important **metabolic** function of bone?

A) Locomotion
B) Protection of vital organs
C) Calcium homeostasis
D) Structural support

14.2. Which of the following terms is used to describe a fibrous connective tissue that connects muscle to bone?

A) Ligament
B) Tendon
C) Synovium
D) Enthesis

14.3. There are numerous anatomical terms related to movement. Which of the following anatomical terms is used to describe movement in the coronal plane **away** from the midline?

A) Adduction
B) Abduction
C) Flexion
D) Extension

14.4. The hip joint is a 'ball and socket' synovial joint, located between the head of the femur and the acetabulum of the innominate (hip) bone. The iliofemoral, pubofemoral and ischiofemoral ligament each contribute to hip stability. Which of the following statements is **true** with regard to these three ligaments that surround the hip joint?

A) The iliofemoral ligament covers the hip joint anteriorly and superiorly, prevents hyperextension of the hip when standing, and is the strongest of the three ligaments
B) The ischiofemoral ligament covers the hip joint anteriorly and inferiorly and prevents excessive abduction
C) The pubofemoral ligament covers the hip joint posteriorly and is the weakest of the three ligaments
D) All of the above

14.5. Which of the following statements is **false** with regard to posterior dislocation of the hip?

A) The sciatic nerve (from spinal cord levels L4-S3) may be injured
B) The limb appears shortened and internally rotated
C) The femoral head is levered out anteriorly
D) Occurs when force is applied to the hip during flexion, internal rotation and adduction

14.6. The knee joint is a hinge synovial joint, composed of three bones. Which of the following bones is **not** associated with the knee joint?

A) Distal femur
B) Proximal tibia
C) Proximal fibula
D) Patella

14.7. Combined knee injury or the 'unhappy triad' occurs due to excessive lateral twisting of a flexed knee or impact to the lateral side of an extended knee. Which of the following structures is **not** part of the 'unhappy triad' of combined knee injury?

A) Tibial (medial) collateral ligament
B) Fibular (lateral) collateral ligament
C) Medial meniscus
D) Anterior cruciate ligament (ACL)

14.8. Osteoarthritis (OA) or wear-and-tear arthritis is a disease of the synovial joints characterised by slowly progressive destruction of the articular cartilage, which impacts upon weight bearing joints and digits. Which of the following is a cardinal **radiological** sign of this degenerative joint disease?

A) Osteophyte formation
B) Subchondral sclerosis and subchondral cyst formation
C) Reduced joint space
D) All of the above

14.9. Which of the following types of muscle fibre are red in colour, very resistant to fatigue and employed in aerobic activities such as long distance running?

A) Type I fibres
B) Type IIa fibres
C) Type IIb fibres
D) None of the above

14.10. The sliding filament model describes the series of events that lead to muscle contraction. Which of the following statements is **false** with regard to this sequence of events?

A) An action potential arrives at the neuromuscular junction (NMJ), resulting in the release of calcium from the sarcoplasmic reticulum
B) Calcium binds to tropomyosin, causing a conformational change and movement of troponin, exposing the myosin-head binding site, so that myosin can attach to actin and form a cross-bridge
C) The hydrolysis of ATP releases energy which drives the repeated attachment, release and re-attachment of myosin heads to actin in a process known as cross-bridge cycling
D) This process repeats itself many times, pulling actin over myosin towards the centre of the sarcomere, so that the whole muscle contracts (shortens)

14.11. Which of the flowing statements is **true** with regard to muscle contraction?

A) During muscle relaxation, there is very little overlap between thin actin filaments and thick myosin filaments
B) The A band moves closer together during muscle contraction
C) The Z lines remain static during muscle contraction
D) None of the above

14.12. Which of the following muscles is **not** a lateral (external) rotator of the hip?

A) Piriformis
B) Gemellus superior
C) Obturator internus
D) Gluteus medius

14.13. Which of the following muscles is an **extensor** of the hip joint and a **flexor** of the knee joint?

A) Semitendinosus
B) Rectus femoris
C) Vastus lateralis
D) Vastus intermedius

14.14. The ankle or talocrural joint is a synovial hinge joint formed by the articulation of the distal tibia and fibula with the talus, which mainly permits two movements: dorsiflexion (extension) and plantarflexion (flexion). Which of the following statements is **true** with regard to dorsiflexion?

A) Dorsiflexion is the most stable position of the ankle joint
B) The muscles responsible for dorsiflexion are located in the anterior compartment of the leg, and supplied by the deep fibular (peroneal) nerve and the anterior tibial artery
C) A and B
D) None of the above

14.15. Inversion and eversion of the foot principally occurs at the subtalar joint, which is located between the talus and calcaneus bones. Which of the following statements is **true** with regard to inversion and eversion injuries of the foot and the ligaments involved?

A) Most ankle sprains are eversion injuries, and occur due to twisting of a plantar-flexed foot
B) The lateral ligament of the ankle is thicker and stronger than the medial (deltoid) ligament
C) A and B
D) None of the above

14.16. The wrist is composed of eight carpal bones, arranged into two rows. From lateral to medial, the distal row includes the trapezium, trapezoid, capitate and hamate, while the proximal row includes the scaphoid, lunate, triquetrum and pisiform. Which of the following is the most commonly fractured carpal bone, often resulting from a fall on an outstretched hand (FOOSH)?

A) Lunate
B) Trapezium
C) Scaphoid
D) Hamate

14.17. The rotator cuff muscles are a group of four short muscles that surround and stabilise the shoulder joint. Which of the following is **not** a rotator cuff muscle?

A) Supraspinatus
B) Infraspinatus
C) Teres major
D) Subscapularis

14.18. The deltoid and supraspinatus muscles are responsible for abduction of the arm. Supraspinatus initiates the first 10-15° of abduction, and then the more powerful deltoid takes over and abducts the arm up to 90°. If a patient's deltoid is paralysed due to anterior dislocation of the shoulder or a fracture of the surgical neck of the humerus, then they are likely to have:

A) Difficulty initiating the first 10-15° of arm abduction
B) Difficulty abducting the arm beyond 15°
C) Damage to the suprascapular nerve
D) All of the above

14.19. Which of the following statements is **true** with regard to the cellular components of bone?

A) Osteoclasts are involved in bone formation and, as such, make osteoid (uncalcified pre-bone tissue) which is mineralised to form bone
B) Osteoblasts are large, multi-nucleated cells that break down bone in a process known as bone resorption
C) Osteoblasts become trapped as osteocytes, which maintain the bone matrix
D) None of the above

14.20. Disordered bone physiology can lead to a great number of metabolic bone diseases. Which of the following metabolic bone diseases has a higher prevalence in men and is characterised by rapid bone turnover and formation, leading to abnormal bone remodelling?

A) Osteoporosis
B) Osteomalacia
C) Paget's disease
D) None of the above

14.21. Loss of bone mass is a characteristic of the natural ageing process in both sexes. Which of the following statements is **false** with regard to ageing and the changes in bone mass that occur in men and women?

A) Peak (maximal) bone mass is reached between 20 and 30 years of age in both males and females
B) The peak bone mass attained in males is higher than in females
C) With increasing age, bone formation increases and bone resorption decreases
D) The rate of bone loss accelerates after the menopause in females

14.22. The elbow is a compound uniaxial synovial joint composed of three bones, which form two closely related articulations. Which of the following three bones form this hinge joint?

A) Humerus, ulna and radius
B) Ulna, clavicle and humerus
C) Distal, intermediate and proximal phalanges
D) Clavicle, scapula and radius

14.23. Which of the following muscles of the upper arm is **not** a flexor of the elbow?

A) Biceps brachii
B) Brachialis
C) Coracobrachialis
D) Brachioradiali

14.24. Patellar dislocation is more common in females than in males. Which of the following statements is **true** with regard to lateral dislocation of the patella?

A) The female pelvis is wider and shallower than the male pelvis
B) The quadriceps angle or Q-angle (the angle at which the femur comes in and aligns with the tibia) is larger in females than in males
C) Lateral dislocation of the patella can occur when the pull of vastus lateralis on the patella overcomes the pull of vastus medialis on the patella
D) All of the above

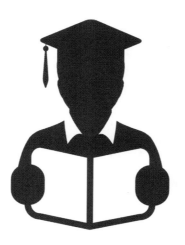

CHAPTER 14

The Musculoskeletal System (MCQs)

Answers and Detailed Solutions

The difficulty rating for each question (Easy, Moderate or Hard) can be found in parentheses next to the correct answer.

14.1. C (Easy)

Bone performs a number of different mechanical functions in the body, including locomotion (movement), structural support and the protection of vital organs (the pelvis, for instance, protects gynaecological and urological organs). In addition, bone is responsible for metabolic functions, such as calcium homeostasis and haematopoiesis (in the bone marrow). Bone functions as a mobilisable store of calcium (and phosphate) and, as such, plays a key role in the homeostatic regulation of these minerals.

14.2. B (Easy)

Tendons and ligaments are fibrous connective tissues that connect muscle to bone and join bone to bone respectively. The enthesis or attachment site is the point where the ligament, tendon, or aponeurosis joins bone. In addition, the synovium or synovial membrane refers to the soft tissue lining the cavities of joints, tendon sheaths and bursae (small fluid-filled sacs that provide a cushion between tendons and bones).

14.3. B (Easy)

There are numerous anatomical terms related to movement. Abduction describes movement in the coronal plane away from the midline, while adduction refers to movement in the coronal plane towards the midline. Extension is a straightening movement (often in the sagittal plane) that increases the angle of a joint. Flexion is a bending movement (often in the sagittal plane) that decreases the angle of a joint.

14.4. A (Hard)

The iliofemoral ligament covers the hip joint anteriorly and superiorly, prevents hyperextension of the hip when standing, and is the strongest of the three ligaments. The pubofemoral ligament covers the hip joint anteriorly and inferiorly and prevents excessive abduction. The ischiofemoral ligament covers the hip joint posteriorly and is the weakest of the three ligaments.

14.5. C (Hard)

Posterior dislocation of the hip occurs when force is applied to the hip during flexion, internal rotation and adduction. Accordingly, it can occur when rising from a seated position or due to the force applied by the dashboard to a seated driver or passenger in a motor vehicle collision. The sciatic nerve (from spinal cord levels L4-S3) may be injured in posterior dislocation, and the limb will appear shortened and internally rotated. Conversely, anterior dislocation occurs when force is applied during substantial abduction with external rotation of the hip. During anterior dislocation, the femoral head is levered out anteriorly, and the limb consequently appears abducted, flexed and externally rotated.

14.6. C (Easy)

The knee joint is a hinge synovial joint, composed of three bones. These include, the distal femur, proximal tibia and the patella. Accordingly, the proximal fibula is not associated with the knee joint.

14.7. B (Hard)

In combined knee injury, ligaments can be injured in isolation or simultaneously. Along these lines, the tibial (medial) collateral ligament tears, followed by the the medial meniscus as these two structures are attached to one another. The anterior cruciate ligament may then also tear, as it is stretched during flexion, and the knee is more vulnerable when flexed than extended, as the knee joint is least stable in flexion.

14.8. D (Moderate)

The four cardinal radiological signs of osteoarthritis (OA) or wear-and-tear arthritis include: osteophyte formation, reduced joint space and subchondral sclerosis and cyst formation. Upon clinical examination, bony swellings, called Heberden's nodes at the distal interphalangeal (DIP) joints and Bouchard's nodes at the proximal interphalangeal (PIP) joints, may also be noted in the hands of individuals with osteoarthritis as a result of osteophyte formation.

CHAPTER 14: The Musculoskeletal System (MCQs)

14.9. A (Moderate)

Slow twitch type I fibres are red in colour due to dense capillaries and high concentrations of myoglobin. They are designed to sustain endurance and, as such, are very resistant to fatigue and contain large amounts of mitochondria. These fibres contract slowly, producing a small amount of power when contracted and are employed in aerobic activities such as long distance running (marathon running). Accordingly, marathon runners will predominately have slow twitch muscle fibres. Fast twitch type II fibres can be divided into type IIa and type IIb fibres. Type IIa fibres (fast twitch A fibres) are red in colour due to high concentrations of myoglobin and resistant to fatigue (albeit not as resistant to fatigue as type I fibres). These fibres contain large amounts of mitochondria and contract relatively quickly, producing a moderate amount of power when contracted. Fast twitch A fibres are used in long-term anaerobic activities such as swimming. Type IIb fibres (fast twitch B fibres) are white in colour due to low concentrations of myoglobin and fatigue very easily. These fibres contain small amounts of mitochondria and contract very quickly, producing a large amount of power when contracted. Fast twitch B fibres are used in short-term anaerobic activities such as sprinting and weightlifting. Sprinters and bodybuilders will thus mainly have fast twitch B fibres.

4.10. B (Hard)

The sliding filament model describes the series of events that lead to muscle contraction. An action potential arrives at the neuromuscular junction (NMJ), resulting in the release of calcium from the sarcoplasmic reticulum. Calcium binds to **troponin**, causing a conformational change and the movement of **tropomyosin**, exposing the myosin-head binding site, so that myosin can attach to actin and form a cross-bridge. The hydrolysis of ATP then releases energy which drives the repeated attachment, release and re-attachment of myosin heads to actin in a process known as cross-bridge cycling. This process repeats itself many times, pulling actin over myosin towards the centre of the sarcomere, so that the whole muscle contracts (shortens).

14.11. A (Hard)

During muscle relaxation, there is very little overlap between thin actin filaments and thick myosin filaments. The Z lines (which anchor the thin actin filaments) move closer together during muscle contraction, while the A band (the entire length of a single thick myosin filament) remains static during muscle contraction.

14.12. D (Moderate)

There are six lateral (external) rotators of the hip: piriformis, gemellus superior, obturator internus, gemellus inferior, quadratus femoris and obturator externus. Conversely, gluteus medius produces abduction and medial rotation at the hip.

14.13. A (Easy)

The hamstring muscles (biceps femoris, semimembranosus and semitendinosus) act as powerful extensors of the hip joint and flexors of the knee joint. In contrast, the quadriceps femoris muscle, which is composed of rectus femoris, vastus lateralis, vastus medialis and vastus intermedius, is a powerful extensor of the knee joint.

14.14. C (Hard)

Dorsiflexion is the most stable position of the ankle joint. The muscles responsible for dorsiflexion are located in the anterior compartment of the leg, and supplied by the deep fibular (peroneal) nerve and the anterior tibial artery. In contrast, the muscles responsible for plantarflexion are located in the posterior compartment of the leg (with the exception of the popliteus muscle), and supplied by the tibial nerve and the posterior tibial artery. Ankle dorsiflexion can be tested by asking a patient to walk around on their heels. Likewise, ankle plantarflexion can be tested by asking a patient to walk around on their tiptoes.

14.15. D (Hard)

Most ankle sprains are inversion (not eversion) injuries, and occur due to twisting of a plantar-flexed foot. This is because the medial (deltoid) ligament of the ankle is thicker and stronger than the lateral ligament. Given that ligaments are relatively avascular structures, the lateral and medial ligaments heal slowly when torn. Torn ligaments can also destabilise the ankle joint and predispose individuals to dislocation.

14.16. C (Easy)

The scaphoid is the most commonly fractured carpal bone. This injury classically results from a fall on an outstretched hand (FOOSH). This is because the scaphoid bone has a narrow 'waist', which leaves it vulnerable to fracture. Scaphoid fracture is a common injury in young adults and is associated with tenderness in a region of the wrist known as the anatomical snuffbox. It can also lead to avascular necrosis, as blood enters the scaphoid distally and then travels proximally. A fracture can thus impair blood supply to the proximal region of the scaphoid bone.

14.17. C (Easy)

The four rotator cuff muscles are the supraspinatus, infraspinatus, teres minor (not teres major) and the subscapularis. Teres major arises from the dorsal surface of the inferior angle of the scapula, and adducts and medially rotates the humerus.

14.18. B (Moderate)

Supraspinatus initiates the first 10-15° of abduction, and then the more powerful deltoid takes over and abducts the arm up to 90°. If a patient's deltoid is paralysed due to anterior dislocation of the shoulder or a fracture of the surgical neck of the humerus, they are thus likely to have difficulty abducting the arm beyond 15°. They will also exhibit damage to the axillary nerve and weakness and atrophy of the deltoid. In contrast, if supraspinatus is paralysed due to, for instance, a scapular fracture, then they will have difficulty initiating the first 10-15° of arm abduction, and there will likely be damage to the suprascapular nerve.

14.19. C (Moderate)

Osteoblasts are involved in bone formation and, as such, make osteoid (uncalcified pre-bone tissue) which is subsequently mineralised to form bone. Osteoclasts are large, multi-nucleated cells that break down bone in a process known as bone resorption. Likewise, osteoblasts become trapped as osteocytes, which maintain the bone matrix.

14.20. C (Moderate)

Paget's disease has a higher prevalence in men and is characterised by rapid bone turnover and formation, leading to abnormal bone remodelling. Osteoporosis is the most common metabolic bone disorder, and is characterised by a generalised decrease in bone mass and microarchitectural deterioration of bone tissue, which leads to fragility of the skeleton and an increased fracture risk. The metabolic disorder osteomalacia (soft bones) is the adult form of childhood rickets, and is associated with inadequate mineralisation of bone matrix (osteoid). It is often caused by insufficient calcium absorption in the intestinal tract, due to vitamin D deficiency. Classic childhood rickets is marked by widened epiphyses and poor skeletal growth.

14.21. C (Moderate)

Peak (maximal) bone mass is reached between 20 and 30 years of age in both males and females. The peak bone mass attained in males is higher than in females. After this peak has been reached, however, at around 50 years of age bone mass starts to decrease with age. Accordingly, with increasing age, bone formation decreases and bone resorption increases. In addition, the rate of bone loss accelerates after the menopause in females.

14.22. A (Easy)

The elbow is a compound uniaxial synovial joint composed of the humerus, ulna and radius. These bones form two closely related articulations: humero-ulnar and humero-radial. The hand is composed of five sets of radiating bones: the carpals (wrist bones) and metacarpals, as well as the proximal, intermediate and distal phalanges. Likewise, the clavicle and scapula form the pectoral (shoulder) girdle.

14.23. C (Moderate)

Biceps brachii, brachialis and brachioradialis all contribute to flexion of the elbow. In contrast, the coracobrachialis is principally associated with forward flexion and adduction of the humerus.

14.24. D (Hard)

The female pelvis is wider and shallower than the male pelvis. Accordingly, the quadriceps angle or Q-angle (the angle at which the femur comes in and aligns with the tibia) is larger in females than in males. This means that, for females, the pull of vastus lateralis on the patella can overcome the pull of vastus medialis. As a result, patellar dislocation is more common in females than in males.

CHAPTER 15
The Nervous System (MCQs)

15.1. The human nervous system is anatomically sub-divided into the central nervous system (CNS) and the peripheral nervous system (PNS). Which of the following structures are located in the **peripheral** nervous system?

A) Brain
B) Spinal Cord
C) Spinal nerves
D) None of the above

15.2. The autonomic nervous system (ANS) has two divisions: sympathetic (adrenergic) and parasympathetic (cholinergic). Activation of the **parasympathetic** nervous system will result in:

A) Pupil dilatation
B) Bronchi dilatation
C) Increased heart rate
D) Increased gut motility

15.3. Each cerebral hemisphere is divided into four functionally distinct lobes: frontal, parietal, occipital and temporal. Which of the following lobes is associated with visual processing and perception?

A) Frontal
B) Parietal
C) Occipital
D) Temporal

15.4. The meninges are three membranous layers that protect and support the brain and spinal cord. From the outermost layer inward, the meninges consist of dura, arachnoid and pia mater. Which of the following statements is **true** with regard to the meninges of the brain?

A) The dura mater consists of two fibrous layers: an internal meningeal layer and an external periosteal layer
B) Arachnoid mater is a soft, translucent membrane, located on the underside of the dura mater
C) Pia mater is a thin, delicate membrane, tightly adhered to the entire surface of the brain
D) All of the above

15.5. Cerebrospinal fluid (CSF) is located between which of the following meningeal layers?

A) Arachnoid and dura
B) Pia and arachnoid
C) A and B
D) None of the above

15.6. Which of the following statements is **false** with regard to the arterial blood supply to the brain?

A) The right and left common carotid arteries bifurcate into the internal and external carotid arteries
B) The external carotid artery (ECA) supplies the brain, while the internal carotid artery (ICA) supplies the face, neck and scalp
C) The vertebral arteries are paired arteries, which originate as branches of the subclavian arteries
D) The vertebral arteries enter the skull via the foramen magnum

15.7. The brainstem connects the spinal cord to the cerebral hemispheres and is composed of three main structures. Which of the following structures is **not** a component of the brainstem?

A) Medulla oblongata
B) Pons
C) Midbrain
D) Hypothalamus

15.8. The cerebellum or little brain is attached to the brainstem via three paired cerebellar peduncles: superior, middle and inferior. Which of the following statements is **false** with regard to the anatomy and function of the cerebellum?

A) The cerebellum coordinates the time, force and duration of muscle action, as well as helping to maintain balance and posture
B) Cerebellar damage can lead to ataxia (uncoordinated movements)
C) The cerebellum is located under the occipital lobes of the cerebral hemispheres, dorsal to the brainstem
D) The cerebellum influences motor coordination on the contralateral side, i.e. the left half of the cerebellum coordinates the action of muscles on the right hand side of the body

15.9. Ten of the twelve pairs of cranial nerves (CNs) arise from the brainstem. Which of the following cranial nerves emerge from the forebrain, not the brainstem?

A) CNs III & IV
B) CNs I & II
C) CNs VII & VIII
D) CNs IX & X

15.10. Which of the following cranial nerves (CNs) emerges from the brainstem at the cerebellopontine angle, passes through the internal acoustic meatus and is associated with hearing and balance?

A) CN VII
B) CN VIII
C) CN IX
D) CN X

15.11. Which of the following cranial nerves (CNs) emerges from the pons, passes through the foramen ovale and provides sensation from the lower face and motor supply to the muscles of mastication?

A) CN III
B) $CN V_1$
C) $CN V_2$
D) $CN V_3$

15.12. Which of the following cranial nerves (CNs) emerges from the anterolateral sulcus (at the junction between the pyramids and olives), passes through the hypoglossal canal and provides motor supply to the muscles of the tongue?

A) CN I
B) CN II
C) CN XI
D) CN XII

15.13. Which of the following cranial nerves (CNs) emerges from the **dorsal** aspect of the brainstem?

A) CN III
B) CN IV
C) CN V
D) CN VI

15.14. There are three classes of myelinated nerve fibre within the white matter of the cerebral hemispheres: association, commissural and projection fibres. Which of the following statements is **true** with regard to these different types of nerve fibre?

A) Association fibres, such as short association fibres, connect cerebral areas within each hemisphere
B) Commissural fibres, such as the corpus callosum, connect the left and right cerebral hemispheres
C) Projection fibres, such as the internal capsule, carry information to and from the cerebral cortex
D) All of the above

15.15. Within the dominant hemisphere, there are two major areas involved in language processing: Broca's and Wernicke's area. Which of the following statements is **false** with regard to these two cortical areas?

A) Broca's area is located in the infero-lateral frontal lobe of the dominant hemisphere, while Wernicke's area is located in the temporal lobe (the posterior part of the superior temporal gyrus) of the dominant hemisphere
B) Wernicke's area is associated with language production and Broca's area is associated with language comprehension
C) Damage to Broca's area can lead to expressive aphasia in which comprehension is largely unimpaired but speech is non-fluent
D) Damage to Wernicke's area can lead to receptive aphasia in which speech is fluent but comprehension is seriously impaired

15.16. The human vertebral column typically consists of 33 spinal vertebrae (cervical, thoracic, lumbar, sacral and coccygeal). How many **thoracic** vertebrae are there in the vertebral column?

A) 5
B) 7
C) 10
D) 12

15.17. There are two types of anaesthesia: general and local (regional). Which of the following statements is **true** with regard to these two major categories of anaesthetic?

A) Local or regional anaesthesia is characterised by total loss of sensation and consciousness
B) General anaesthesia is characterised by loss of sensation to a particular region or part of the body
C) Local or regional anaesthetic agents work by reversibly preventing the transmission of a nerve impulse to a particular region or part of the body, without affecting consciousness
D) All anaesthetic agents produce the following three neurobiological effects: amnesia, hypnosis and immobility

15.18. The accommodation reflex is a series of changes that occur when the focus of the eyes shifts from a distant object to a near object. Which of the following changes does **not** take place as part of this reflex?

A) Contraction of the ciliary muscles
B) Contraction of the medial rectus extraocular muscles
C) Contraction of the lateral rectus extraocular muscles
D) Pupillary constriction (miosis)

15.19. The pupillary light reflex refers to the ability of both pupils to respond (constrict or dilate) to light as it is received by the retina. Which of the following statements is **false** with regard to this reflex?

A) A light is shone into one eye and the pupil in that eye constricts in the direct light reflex
B) A light is shone into one eye and the pupil in the other eye constricts in the consensual light reflex
C) The sensory (afferent) root of this reflex is the oculomotor nerve (CN III) and the motor (efferent) root of this reflex is the optic nerve (CN II) and tract
D) All of the above

15.20. There are two types of photoreceptor in the retina at the back of the eye: cones (associated with colour vision) and rods (associated with black and white vision). Which of the following statements is **false** with regard to the differences between these two photoreceptors?

A) Rods have a high sensitivity to light and are therefore specialised for night vision
B) Cones have a low sensitivity to light and are therefore specialised for day vision
C) Cones have low visual acuity and are not present in the fovea, while rods have high visual acuity and are concentrated in the fovea at the centre of the retina
D) All of the above

15.21. Visual field defects can be caused by injury to any point along the visual pathway, from the retina to the cerebral cortex. Which of the following terms is used to describe visual pathway damage if **half** of the visual field is lost?

A) Scotoma
B) Anopia
C) Hemianopia
D) Quadrantanopia

15.22. The middle ear lies within the temporal bone of the skull and contains three bony ossicles: the malleus (hammer), incus (anvil) and stapes (stirrup). Which of the following statements is **true** with regard to these auditory ossicles?

A) Sound waves hit the tympanic membrane (TM) or eardrum, causing it to vibrate and set the malleus, incus and stapes in motion, which converts sound energy into mechanical energy
B) The bony ossicles are the smallest bones in the human body
C) A and B
D) None of the above

15.23. There are two common types of deafness: conductive and sensorineural. Which of the following statements is **true** with regard to these two types of hearing impairment?

A) Conductive deafness is a defect of sound transmission up to the spiral ganglion, while sensorineural deafness is a defect in the function of the spiral ganglion or the cochlear nerve
B) A patient with sensorineural deafness will be deaf to ordinary air conduction but display no deafness to bone conduction
C) A patient with conductive deafness will be deaf to both air and bone conduction
D) All of the above

15.24. The Weber's and Rinne tests can be employed to determine whether a patient has sensorineural or conductive hearing loss. Which of the following statements is **false** with regard to the interpretation of these tuning fork tests?

A) In Weber's test, the patient will hear the tuning fork louder in the damaged ear if they have conductive hearing loss
B) In Weber's test, the tuning fork will be better heard by the patient in the normal ear if they have sensorineural hearing loss
C) In Rinne's test, the patient will hear bone conduction and air conduction for an equal length of time if they have conductive hearing loss
D) In Rinne's test, the patient will hear air conduction for longer than bone conduction if they have sensorineural hearing loss

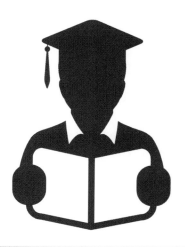

CHAPTER 15

The Nervous System (MCQs)

Answers and Detailed Solutions

The difficulty rating for each question (Easy, Moderate or Hard) can be found in parentheses next to the correct answer.

15.1. C (Easy)

The central nervous system (CNS) comprises the brain and the spinal cord, which are enclosed in the skull and the vertebral column respectively. Radiating away from the CNS, is the peripheral nervous system (PNS). The PNS consists of the peripheral nerves, which emerge from the brain (cranial nerves) and the spinal cord (spinal nerves). The PNS can be functionally divided into the somatic nervous system (SNS) and the autonomic nervous system (ANS).

15.2. D (Easy)

Activation of the parasympathetic nervous system (the rest-and-digest response) will result in increased gut motility. In contrast, activation of the sympathetic nervous system (the fight-or-flight response) will result in pupil dilatation, bronchi dilatation and an increased heart rate. Along these lines, the sympathetic and parasympathetic nervous systems tend to have opposing physiological effects.

15.3. C (Easy)

The frontal lobe is associated with reasoning, judgement and decision making, as well as skilled voluntary movements, while the parietal lobe is concerned with visuospatial localisation and perception of the body. Likewise, the temporal lobe is associated with auditory perception, cognition and memory, while the occipital lobe is important for visual processing and perception.

15.4. D (Moderate)

From the outermost layer inward, the meninges consists of dura, arachnoid and pia mater. The dura mater consists of two fibrous layers: an internal meningeal layer and an external periosteal layer. Arachnoid mater is a soft, translucent membrane, located on the underside of the dura mater. Pia mater is a thin, delicate membrane, tightly adhered to the entire surface of the brain.

15.5. B (Easy)

The subarachnoid space lies between the pia and the arachnoid mater, and contains cerebrospinal fluid (CSF). Cerebrospinal fluid serves to cushion, protect and nourish the brain and the spinal cord. The subdural space is a potential space that lies between the arachnoid and the dura mater. If a skull fracture penetrates into the subarachnoid space then cerebrospinal fluid may leak out. Similarly, if cerebrospinal fluid circulation is blocked in the ventricular system, it can accumulate upstream of the blockage leading to hydrocephalus.

15.6. B (Moderate)

The right and left common carotid arteries bifurcate into the internal and external carotid arteries. The internal carotid artery (ICA) supplies the brain, while the external carotid artery (ECA) supplies the face, neck and scalp. In like manner, the vertebral arteries are paired arteries, which originate as branches of the subclavian arteries and enter the skull via the foramen magnum.

15.7. D (Easy)

The brainstem is composed of the medulla oblongata, pons and midbrain. The medulla oblongata is continuous caudally with the spinal cord at the level of the foramen magnum, while the midbrain is continuous rostrally with the diencephalon. The diencephalon is composed of the thalamus, epithalamus, hypothalamus and subthalamus and, as such, the hypothalamus is not a component of the brainstem. The hypothalamus is composed of several nuclei and has autonomic and neuroendocrine functions.

15.8. D (Hard)

The cerebellum or little brain coordinates the time, force and duration of muscle action, as well as helping to maintain balance and posture. Accordingly, cerebellar damage can lead to ataxia (uncoordinated movements). The cerebellum influences motor coordination on the **ipsilateral** side, i.e. the left half of the cerebellum coordinates the action of muscles on the left hand side of the body. In addition, the cerebellum is located under the occipital lobes of the cerebral hemispheres, dorsal to the brainstem.

15.9. B (Moderate)

The olfactory and optic nerve (CNs I & II respectively) are not typical cranial nerves as they emerge from the forebrain, not the brainstem. In contrast, CNs III (the oculomotor nerve), IV (the trochlear nerve), V (the trigeminal nerve), VI (the abducens nerve), VII (the facial nerve), VIII (the vestibulocochlear nerve), IX (the glossopharyngeal nerve), X (the vagus nerve), XI (the accessory nerve) and XII (the hypoglossal nerve) arise from the brainstem.

15.10. B (Hard)

The vestibulocochlear nerve (CN VIII) emerges from the brainstem at the cerebellopontine angle, passes through the internal acoustic meatus and is associated with hearing and balance. The facial nerve (CN VII) also emerges from the brainstem at the cerebellopontine angle, passes through the internal acoustic meatus and provides motor function to the muscles of facial expression, parasympathetic supply to all major and minor glands of the head (except the parotid gland) and conveys taste sensation from the anterior 2/3^{rds} of the tongue. The glossopharyngeal nerve (CN IX) emerges from the posterolateral sulcus of the medulla (lateral to the olives), passes through the jugular foramen and provides parasympathetic supply to the parotid gland, cutaneous sensation from the ear and sensation from the carotid body. In addition, it conveys taste sensation from the posterior 1/3rd of the tongue and assists with swallowing. Likewise, the vagus nerve (CN X) emerges from the posterolateral sulcus of the medulla (lateral to the olives), passes through the jugular foramen and provides sensory and motor supply to the muscles of the pharynx and larynx and parasympathetic innervation to all thoracic viscera and the gastrointestinal (GI) tract. It also carries taste sensation from the epiglottis and palate.

15.11. D (Hard)

The oculomotor nerve (CN III) emerges from the brainstem at the pontomesencephalic junction in the interpeduncular fossa, passes through the superior orbital fissure and supplies four of the six extraocular muscles. The ophthalmic division of the trigeminal nerve (CN V_1) emerges from the pons, passes through the superior orbital fissure and provides sensation from the upper face. The maxillary division of the trigeminal nerve (CN V_2) emerges from the pons, passes through the foramen rotundum and provides sensation from the middle face. The mandibular division of the trigeminal nerve (CN V_3) emerges from the pons, passes through the foramen ovale and provides sensation from the lower face and motor supply to the muscles of mastication.

15.12. D (Hard)

The hypoglossal nerve (CN XII) emerges from the anterolateral sulcus (at the junction between the pyramids and olives), passes through the hypoglossal canal and provides motor supply to the muscles of the tongue. The accessory nerve (CN XI) emerges caudal to the medulla and rostral to the spinal cord, passes through the jugular foramen and supplies motor innervation to the sternocleidomastoid (SCM) and the trapezius muscles. The olfactory nerve (CN I) and the optic nerve (CN II) emerge from the forebrain, and are associated with smell (olfaction) and vision respectively.

15.13. B (Moderate)

The trochlear nerve (CN IV) is the only cranial nerve that emerges from the dorsal aspect of the brainstem (the dorsal midbrain). This nerve passes through the superior orbital fissure and supplies the superior oblique extraocular muscle. The abducens nerve (CN VI) emerges at the pontomedullary junction, passes through the superior orbital fissure and supplies the lateral rectus extraocular muscle. For further information about the oculomotor nerve (CN III) and the trigeminal nerve (CN V) refer to the detailed solution for question 15.11. in this chapter.

15.14. D (Hard)

Association fibres, such as short association fibres, connect cerebral areas within each hemisphere while commissural fibres, such as the corpus callosum, connect the left and right cerebral hemispheres. In like manner, projection fibres, such as the internal capsule, carry information to and from the cerebral cortex.

15.15. B (Moderate)

Broca's area is located in the infero-lateral frontal lobe of the dominant hemisphere, while Wernicke's area is located in the temporal lobe (the posterior part of the superior temporal gyrus) of the dominant hemisphere. Broca's area is associated with language production and Wernicke's area is associated with language comprehension. Along these lines, damage to Broca's area can lead to expressive aphasia in which comprehension is largely unimpaired but speech is non-fluent. In like manner, damage to Wernicke's area can lead to receptive aphasia in which speech is fluent but comprehension is seriously impaired.

15.16. D (Easy)

The human vertebral column typically consists of 33 spinal vertebrae: 7 cervical, 12 thoracic, 5 lumbar, 5 sacral and 4 coccygeal.

15.17. C (Moderate)

General anaesthesia is characterised by total loss of sensation and consciousness, while local or regional anaesthesia is characterised by loss of sensation to a particular region or part of the body. Local or regional anaesthetic agents work by reversibly preventing the transmission of a nerve impulse to a particular region or part of the body, without affecting consciousness. Along these lines, the neurobiological effects of anaesthetic agents include amnesia, hypnosis and immobility, however, not all anaesthetics will produce all three of these effects.

15.18. C (Moderate)

During the accommodation reflex, the lens becomes rounded and thicker due to contraction of the ciliary muscles. This ensures that the image is focused on the retina. Likewise, the medial rectus extraocular muscles contract and the lateral rectus extraocular muscles relax. This adducts the eyes and helps to ensure that the object is directly focused onto the fovea as it approaches (ocular convergence). Pupillary constriction (miosis) also occurs in order to increase the depth of focus.

15.19. C (Moderate)

Two cranial nerves (CNs) are associated with the pupillary light reflex. The sensory (afferent) root of this reflex is the optic nerve (CN II) and tract, and the motor (efferent) root of this reflex is the oculomotor nerve (CN III). In the direct light reflex, a light is shone into one eye and the pupil in that eye constricts. Similarly, in the consensual light reflex, a light is shone into one eye and the pupil in the other eye constricts.

15.20. C (Easy)

Rods have a high sensitivity to light and are therefore specialised for night vision. In contrast, cones have a low sensitivity to light and are therefore specialised for day vision. Rods have low visual acuity and are not present in the fovea, while cones have high visual acuity and are concentrated in the fovea at the centre of the retina.

15.21. C (Hard)

A scotoma is a localised patch of blindness within the visual field, while anopia or anopsia denotes the loss of one or more quadrants of the visual field. Hemianopia or hemianopsia describes loss of half of the visual field. Likewise, quadrantanopia or quadrantanopsia refers to loss in a quarter (quadrant) of the visual field. Visual field losses affect the same side of the visual field in each eye in homonymous defects. Similarly, visual field losses affect opposite sides of the visual field in each eye in heteronymous defects.

15.22. C (Easy)

Sound waves hit the tympanic membrane (TM) or eardrum, causing it to vibrate and set the malleus (hammer), incus (anvil) and stapes (stirrup) in motion, which converts sound energy into mechanical energy. These bony or auditory ossicles are the smallest bones in the human body.

15.23. A (Hard)

Conductive deafness is a defect of sound transmission up to the spiral ganglion, while sensorineural deafness is a defect in the function of the spiral ganglion or the cochlear nerve. Along these lines, a patient with conductive deafness will be deaf to ordinary air conduction but display no deafness to bone conduction. Likewise, a patient with sensorineural deafness will be deaf to both air and bone conduction.

15.24. C (Hard)

In Weber's test, the patient will hear the tuning fork louder in the damaged ear if they have conductive hearing loss. Likewise, in sensorineural hearing loss, the tuning fork will be better heard by the patient in the normal ear. In Rinne's test, the patient will hear bone conduction for longer than air conduction if they have conductive hearing loss. Similarly, in sensorineural hearing loss, the patient will hear air conduction for longer than bone conduction.

CHAPTER 16
Public Health (EMQs)

Theme

Epidemiology

Options

- **A)** Incidence
- **B)** Lead-time bias
- **C)** Length-time bias
- **D)** Negative predictive value (NPV)
- **E)** Point prevalence
- **F)** Positive predictive value (PPV)
- **G)** Sensitivity
- **H)** Specificity

Instructions

For each question in the list below (16.1.-16.6.), choose the single most appropriate answer from the list above (A-H). Each option may be used once, more than once or not at all.

Questions

16.1. The probability that someone with a positive test result actually has the disease

16.2. The number of new cases of a disease over a specific period of time

16.3. The number of people with a given disease at a particular date in time

16.4. The proportion of people who actually have the disease and are correctly identified by a positive test result

16.5. Screening over-represents the less aggressive disease

16.6. The probability that someone with a negative test result does not actually have the disease

Theme

Study Designs

Options

- **A)** Case control study
- **B)** Case series
- **C)** Cohort study
- **D)** Cross-sectional study
- **E)** Ecological study
- **F)** Mendelian randomisation (MR)
- **G)** Meta-analysis (MA)
- **H)** Randomised controlled trial (RCT)

Instructions

For each question in the list below (16.7.-16.12.), choose the single most appropriate answer from the list above (A-H). Each option may be used once, more than once or not at all.

Questions

16.7. The unit of observation is a group (such as a population, country or region), not an individual

16.8. A snapshot of a defined population with an outcome at a specific point in time

16.9. A retrospective observational study in which cases and controls are compared with respect to previous exposure status

16.10. A prospective observational study in which people who share a common experience are followed through time for an outcome

16.11. Participants are randomly allocated to a treatment group or a control group and then followed through time to determine who develops the disease outcome

16.12. A type of systematic review in which the results of various independent studies are combined and integrated in order to help answer a specific research problem

CHAPTER 16: Public Health (EMQs)

Theme

Quantifying risk

Options

- A) Absolute risk
- B) Absolute risk reduction (ARR)
- C) Attributable risk (AR)
- D) Number needed to harm (NNH)
- E) Number needed to treat (NNT)
- F) Odds ratio (OR)
- G) Relative risk (RR)
- H) Relative risk reduction (RRR)

Instructions

For each question in the list below (16.13.-16.18.), choose the single most appropriate answer from the list above (A-H). Each option may be used once, more than once or not at all.

Questions

16.13. The probability that a person experiences a specified event
16.14. The ratio of absolute risks among exposed individuals compared to non-exposed individuals
16.15. 1 – Relative risk (RR)
16.16. Event rate in intervention group – Event rate in control group
16.17. The number of people who would need to receive a treatment in order for one of them to experience an adverse effect
16.18. The number of people who would need to receive a treatment in order for one of them to derive a benefit

Theme

Statistics

Options

- **A)** Confidence interval (CI)
- **B)** Mean
- **C)** P-value (probability value)
- **D)** Reliability
- **E)** Responsiveness
- **F)** Standard deviation (SD)
- **G)** Standard error (SE)
- **H)** Validity

Instructions

For each question in the list below (16.19.-16.24.), choose the single most appropriate answer from the list above (A-H). Each option may be used once, more than once or not at all.

Questions

16.19. The range within which you can be 95% certain that the real answer lies

16.20. The probability that the results have arisen due to chance

16.21. The ability of an instrument to detect real changes when they occur

16.22. The extent to which an instrument measures accurately what it is meant to measure

16.23. The extent to which an instrument gives the same result on retesting

16.24. A measure of spread

CHAPTER 16

Public Health (EMQs)

Answers and Detailed Solutions

The difficulty rating for each question (Easy, Moderate or Hard) can be found in parentheses next to the correct answer.

16.1. F (Moderate)
16.2. A (Easy)
16.3. E (Easy)
16.4. G (Moderate)
16.5. C (Hard)
16.6. D (Moderate)

Sensitivity, specificity, positive predictive value (PPV) and negative predictive value (NPV) are four key measures used in the evaluation of diagnostic test performance. Positive predictive value (PPV) is the probability that someone with a positive test result actually has the disease, while negative predictive value (NPV) is the probability that someone with a negative test result does not actually have the disease. Sensitivity is the proportion of people who actually have the disease and are correctly identified by a positive test result. Specificity is the proportion of people who do not have the disease and are correctly re-assured by a negative test result. In essence, sensitivity tells you how well a test detects individuals with the disease, and specificity tells you how well a test correctly excludes individuals without the disease. Incidence and prevalence provide measures of disease frequency. Incidence refers to the number of **new** cases of a disease over a specific period of time. In contrast, prevalence denotes the number of people with a given disease at a particular date in time (point prevalence) or during a specified period of time (period prevalence). Lead-time bias and length-time bias are potential biases in screening evaluation. Length-time bias is used to describe how screening over-represents the less aggressive disease, while lead-time bias occurs when early diagnosis falsely appears to prolong survival.

16.7. E (Easy)
16.8. D (Easy)
16.9. A (Moderate)
16.10. C (Moderate)
16.11. H (Moderate)
16.12. G (Hard)

A cross-sectional study provides a snapshot of a defined population with an outcome at a specific point in time. This study design is primarily used to measure disease prevalence. A case-control study is a retrospective study in which cases (people with the disease) and controls (people without the disease) are compared with respect to previous exposure status, for example people with and without lung cancer are interviewed about their smoking history. Conversely, a cohort study is a prospective observational study in which people who share a common experience are followed through time for an outcome. In ecological studies the unit of observation is a group (such as a population, country or region), not an individual. Randomised controlled trials (RCTs) are considered to be the 'gold standard' of medical research, while descriptive studies, such as case series are regarded as the weakest study design. In a randomised controlled trial (RCT), participants are randomly allocated to a treatment group or a control group and then followed through time to determine who develops the disease outcome. A meta-analysis (MA) is a type of systematic review in which the results of various independent studies are combined and integrated in order to help answer a specific research problem. Mendelian randomisation (MR) is an observational design, in which a genetic variant is used as a proxy for an exposure.

16.13. A (Easy)
16.14. G (Hard)
16.15. H (Hard)
16.16. B (Hard)
16.17. D (Easy)
16.18. E (Easy)

Absolute risk describes the probability that a person experiences a specified event. Relative risk (or comparative risk) is the ratio of absolute risks among exposed individuals compared to non-exposed individuals. The odds ratio (OR) is similar to relative risk, except that it refers to a ratio of odds rather than a ratio of risks. Absolute risk reduction (or risk difference) is the simple difference in event rate between the control and the treatment group, while the relative risk reduction (RRR) sets out the relative difference between the two event rates. Attributable risk (AR) represents the excess risk of disease due to exposure in the exposed group. Number needed to harm (NNH) denotes the number of people who would need to receive a treatment in order for one of them to experience an adverse effect. Conversely, number needed to treat (NNT) is the number

CHAPTER 16: Public Health (EMQs)

of people who would need to receive a treatment in order for one of them to derive a benefit.

The following equations can be used when quantifying risk:

$$\text{Relative risk (RR)} = \frac{\text{Event rate in intervention group}}{\text{Event rate in control group}}$$

$$\text{Relative risk reduction (RRR)} = 1 - \text{Relative risk} \text{ or } \frac{\text{Absolute risk reduction}}{\text{Event rate in control group}}$$

Absolute risk reduction (ARR) = Event rate in intervention group - Event rate in control group

$$\text{Number needed to harm (NNH)} = \frac{1}{\text{Attributable risk}}$$

$$\text{Number needed to treat (NNT)} = \frac{1}{\text{Absolute risk reduction}}$$

16.19. A (Moderate)
16.20. C (Moderate)
16.21. E (Hard)
16.22. H (Hard)
16.23. D (Hard)
16.24. F (Easy)

The p-value (probability value) expresses the probability that the results have arisen due to chance. A p-value of <0.05 is considered to be statistically significant, as there is a very small probability that the results have arisen due to chance. The confidence interval (CI) is the range within which you can be 95% certain that the real answer lies. A narrow confidence interval indicates a more precise estimate and vice-versa. High quality outcome measures should be valid, responsive and reliable. Validity refers to the extent to which an instrument measures accurately what it is meant to measure, while responsiveness denotes the ability of an instrument to detect real changes when they occur. Likewise, reliability describes the extent to which an instrument gives the same result on retesting. Standard deviation (SD) is a measure of spread, standard error (SE) is a measure of precision and the mean (along with the median and the mode) is a measure of location.

CHAPTER 17
Pharmacology and Therapeutics I (EMQs)

Theme

Cardiovascular pharmacology

Options

- A) Atropine
- B) Adenosine
- C) Digoxin
- D) Simvastatin and atorvastatin
- E) Verapamil and diltiazem
- F) Losartan and valsartan
- G) Amlodipine and nifedipine
- H) Enalapril and ramipril

Instructions

For each question in the list below (17.1.-17.6.), choose the single most appropriate answer from the list above (A-H). Each option may be used once, more than once or not at all.

Questions

17.1. Dihydropyridine calcium channel blockers (DHPCCBs), which have a high ratio of vascular to cardiac selectivity

17.2. Non-dihydropyridine calcium channel blockers (non-DHPCCBs), which have a low ratio of vascular to cardiac selectivity

17.3. Angiotensin-converting-enzyme inhibitors (ACEi), which inhibit the conversion of angiotensin I (Ang I) to angiotensin II (Ang II)

17.4. Angiotensin II receptor blockers (ARBs), which inhibit the binding of angiotensin II (Ang II) to the angiotensin II type 1 (AT1) receptor

17.5. A cardiac glycoside, which can cause xanthopsia (yellowish visual discolouration) and 'reverse tick' ST depression on an electrocardiogram (ECG)

17.6. Lipid lowering agents, which reduce blood cholesterol levels by inhibiting the enzyme 3-hydroxy-3-methylglutaryl-coenzyme A (HMG-CoA) reductase

Theme

Respiratory pharmacology

Options

A) Beclomethasone
B) Ipratropium bromide
C) Salbutamol
D) Salmeterol
E) Prednisolone
F) Montelukast
G) Tiotropium
H) Theophylline

Instructions

For each question in the list below (17.7.-17.12.), choose the single most appropriate answer from the list above (A-H). Each option may be used once, more than once or not at all.

Questions

17.7. A short-acting β_2-agonist, which is given by metered-dose inhaler (MDI) and is active for up to four hours after inhalation

17.8. A long-acting β_2-agonist, which is given by metered-dose inhaler (MDI) and is active for up to twelve hours after inhalation

17.9. A leukotriene receptor antagonist (LTRA)

17.10. A methylxanthine

17.11. A short-acting muscarinic antagonist (SAMA), which is used in the management of chronic obstructive pulmonary disease (COPD)

17.12. A long-acting muscarinic antagonist (LAMA), which is used in the management of chronic obstructive pulmonary disease (COPD)

CHAPTER 17: Pharmacology and Therapeutics I (EMQs)

Theme

Blood glucose-lowering therapy in type II diabetes mellitus

Options

A) Thiazolidinediones (TZDs) or glitazones, such as pioglitazone
B) Biguanides, such as metformin
C) Glucagon-like peptide-1 receptor agonists (GLP-1 RAs), such as exenatide and liraglutide
D) Sodium-glucose co-transporter-2 inhibitors (SGLT-2i), such as canagliflozin and dapagliflozin
E) Dipeptidyl peptidase-4 (DPP-4) inhibitors or gliptins, such as sitagliptin and vildagliptin
F) Sulfonylureas, such as gliclazide and glibenclamide
G) α-glucosidase inhibitors (AGIs), such as acarbose
H) Meglitinides, such as nateglinide and repaglinide

Instructions

For each question in the list below (17.13.-17.18.), choose the single most appropriate answer from the list above (A-H). Each option may be used once, more than once or not at all.

Questions

17.13. First-line oral anti-diabetic drugs (OADs), which increase peripheral insulin sensitivity and decrease hepatic gluconeogenesis
17.14. Second or third line oral anti-diabetic drugs (OADs), which stimulate the endogenous release of insulin from pancreatic β cells
17.15. Second or third line oral anti-diabetic drugs (OADs), which reduce glucose reabsorption in the kidneys
17.16. Synthetic ligands for peroxisome proliferator-activated receptor gamma (PPARγ), which increase peripheral insulin sensitisation and affect lipid metabolism
17.17. Second or third line oral anti-diabetic drugs (OADs), which increase insulin secretion and inhibit glucagon secretion
17.18. Fourth line anti-diabetic drugs, often administered subcutaneously, which increase insulin secretion and inhibit glucagon secretion

Theme

Renal pharmacology

Options

A) Furosemide and bumetanide
B) Indapamide and chlorthalidone
C) Bendroflumethiazide and hydrochlorothiazide
D) Acetazolamide (AZ)
E) Spironolactone
F) Amiloride
G) Mannitol
H) Empagliflozin

Instructions

For each question in the list below (17.19.-17.24.), choose the single most appropriate answer from the list above (A-H). Each option may be used once, more than once or not at all.

Questions

17.19. Thiazide diuretics, which inhibit the reabsorption of sodium in the early distal convoluted tubule (DCT), by blocking the sodium-chloride symporter

17.20. Loop diuretics, which inhibit the activity of the sodium-potassium-chloride cotransporter in the thick ascending loop of Henle (TALH), thereby reducing the absorption of sodium chloride

17.21. Thiazide-like diuretics, which are used in the treatment of hypertension

17.22. A carbonic anhydrase inhibitor (CAI), which can be used in the treatment of glaucoma as it reduces intraocular pressure (IOP)

17.23. An osmotic diuretic, which is used in the treatment of cerebral oedema

17.24. A mineralocorticoid receptor antagonist (MRA), which can cause hyperkalaemia and gynecomastia

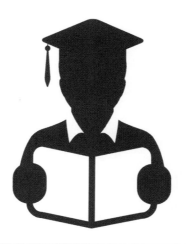

CHAPTER 17

Pharmacology and Therapeutics I (EMQs)

Answers and Detailed Solutions

The difficulty rating for each question (Easy, Moderate or Hard) can be found in parentheses next to the correct answer.

17.1. G (Hard)
17.2. E (Hard)
17.3. H (Easy)
17.4. F (Easy)
17.5. C (Hard)
17.6. D (Moderate)

Amlodipine and nifedipine are dihydropyridine calcium channel blockers (DHPCCBs). These peripheral vasodilators have a high ratio of vascular to cardiac selectivity, and as such, are commonly used to lower blood pressure (BP). In contrast, verapamil and diltiazem are non-dihydropyridine calcium channel blockers (non-DHPCCBs). These cardioselective agents have a low ratio of vascular to cardiac selectivity, and are thus often used to reduce cardiac contractility and heart rate (HR). Enalapril and ramipril are examples of angiotensin-converting-enzyme inhibitors (ACEi), which inhibit the conversion of angiotensin I (Ang I) to angiotensin II (Ang II). Losartan and valsartan are examples of angiotensin II receptor blockers (ARBs), which inhibit the binding of angiotensin II to the angiotensin II type 1 (AT_1) receptor. Digoxin is a cardiac glycoside, which can cause xanthopsia (yellowish visual discolouration) and 'reverse tick' ST depression on an electrocardiogram (ECG). Simvastatin and atorvastatin are lipid lowering agents (statins), which reduce blood cholesterol levels by inhibiting the enzyme 3-hydroxy-3-methylglutaryl-coenzyme A (HMG-CoA) reductase. Adenosine is an endogenous nucleoside, which can be used in the diagnosis and treatment of supraventricular tachycardia (SVT), while atropine is commonly used for the treatment of bradycardia.

17.7. C (Easy)
17.8. D (Easy)
17.9. F (Moderate)
17.10. H (Moderate)
17.11. B (Easy)
17.12. G (Easy)

Salbutamol is a short-acting β_2-agonist, which is given by metered-dose inhaler (MDI) and is active for up to four hours after inhalation. Salmeterol is a long-acting β_2-agonist, which is given by metered-dose inhaler and is active for up to twelve hours after inhalation. The latter two bronchodilators are both used in the management of chronic asthma and chronic obstructive pulmonary disease (COPD). Montelukast (a leukotriene receptor antagonist [LTRA]) and theophylline (a methylxanthine) are also bronchodilators. In contrast to theophylline, however, which is used in the management of chronic asthma and COPD, montelukast is not used in the management of COPD. Ipratropium bromide (a short-acting muscarinic antagonist [SAMA]) and tiotropium (a long-acting muscarinic antagonist [LAMA]), are used in the management of COPD. Beclomethasone is an inhaled corticosteroid (ICS), which is often given in low doses in the management of chronic asthma. Prednisolone is a systemic steroid, which is commonly given during acute exacerbations of asthma and COPD.

17.13. B (Moderate)
17.14. F (Moderate)
17.15. D (Hard)
17.16. A (Hard)
17.17. E (Hard)
17.18. C (Hard)

Biguanides, such as metformin are first-line oral anti-diabetic drugs (OADs), which increase peripheral insulin sensitivity and decrease hepatic gluconeogenesis. Sulfonylureas, such as gliclazide and glibenclamide are second or third line oral anti-diabetic drugs, which stimulate the endogenous release of insulin from pancreatic β cells. Thiazolidinediones (TZDs) or glitazones, such as pioglitazone are synthetic ligands for peroxisome proliferator-activated receptor gamma (PPARγ), which increase peripheral insulin sensitisation and affect lipid metabolism. Sodium-glucose co-transporter-2 inhibitors (SGLT-2i), such as canagliflozin and dapagliflozin are second or third line oral anti-diabetic drugs, which reduce glucose reabsorption in the kidneys. Dipeptidyl peptidase-4 (DPP-4) inhibitors or gliptins, such as sitagliptin and vildagliptin are second or third line oral anti-diabetic drugs, which increase insulin secretion and inhibit glucagon secretion. Glucagon-like peptide-1 receptor agonists (GLP-1 RAs), such as exenatide and liraglutide, are fourth line anti-diabetic drugs, often administered subcutaneously, which increase insulin secretion and inhibit glucagon secretion. Starch blockers or α-glucosidase inhibitors (AGIs), such as acarbose, are oral anti-diabetic drugs, which decrease the rate at which complex carbohydrates are digested and thus reduce post-prandial hyperglycaemia. Finally, meglitinides, such as nateglinide and repaglinide, are oral anti-diabetic drugs, which stimulate the endogenous release of insulin from pancreatic β cells in a similar manner to sulfonylureas.

17.19. C (Easy)
17.20. A (Easy)
17.21. B (Moderate)
17.22. D (Moderate)
17.23. G (Hard)
17.24. E (Moderate)

Bendroflumethiazide and hydrochlorothiazide are thiazide diuretics, which inhibit the reabsorption of sodium in the early distal convoluted tubule (DCT), by blocking the sodium-chloride symporter. Similarly, furosemide and bumetanide are loop diuretics, which inhibit the activity of the sodium-potassium-chloride cotransporter in the thick ascending limb of the loop of Henle (TALH), thereby reducing the absorption of sodium chloride. Indapamide and chlorthalidone are thiazide-like diuretics, used in the treatment of hypertension. Acetazolamide (AZ) is a carbonic anhydrase inhibitor (CAI), which can be used in the treatment of glaucoma as it reduces intraocular pressure (IOP). Spironolactone is a mineralocorticoid receptor antagonist (MRA), which can cause hyperkalaemia and gynecomastia. Amiloride is also a potassium-sparing diuretic, unlike spironolactone however it does not cause gynecomastia. Mannitol is an osmotic diuretic, which is used in the treatment of cerebral oedema. Empagliflozin is a sodium-glucose co-transporter-2 inhibitor (SGLT-2i), and a second or third line oral anti-diabetic drug (OAD), which reduces glucose reabsorption in the kidneys.

CHAPTER 18
Pharmacology and Therapeutics II (EMQs)

Theme

Pharmacology of the endocrine system

Options

A) Amiodarone
B) Intravenous (IV) calcium gluconate
C) Nebulised (neb) salbutamol
D) Octreotide
E) Levothyroxine
F) Dextrose and insulin infusion
G) Phenoxybenzamine followed by propranolol
H) Carbimazole

Instructions

For each question in the list below (18.1.-18.6.), choose the single most appropriate answer from the list above (A-H). Each option may be used once, more than once or not at all.

Questions

18.1. A somatostatin analogue, used for the medical management of acromegaly
18.2. An antiarrhythmic drug, which can precipitate both hyperthyroidism and hypothyroidism
18.3. The first-line drug in the emergency treatment of hyperkalaemia
18.4. The medical management of a phaeochromocytoma
18.5. A drug treatment for thyrotoxicosis, which can cause agranulocytosis (a low white blood cell count) in rare cases
18.6. A synthetic thyroid hormone used for the treatment of hypothyroidism

Theme

Gastrointestinal (GI) pharmacology

Options

A) Cinnarizine and cyclizine
B) Omeprazole and lansoprazole
C) Ondansetron and granisetron
D) Terlipressin
E) Loperamide
F) N-acetylcysteine (NAC)
G) Prednisolone
H) Penicillamine

Instructions

For each question in the list below (18.7.-18.12.), choose the single most appropriate answer from the list above (A-H). Each option may be used once, more than once or not at all.

Questions

18.7. Proton pump inhibitors (PPIs), which reduce gastric acid secretion by irreversibly inhibiting the hydrogen-potassium ATPase enzyme system in gastric parietal cells

18.8. 5-hydroxytryptamine type 3 (5-HT$_3$) receptor antagonists, most commonly used for the prevention of chemotherapy-induced nausea and vomiting (N&V)

18.9. Antihistamines (H$_1$-receptor antagonists), which have antiemetic properties and can be used to treat Ménière's disease (a rare disorder characterised by vertigo, hearing loss and tinnitus)

18.10. An anti-motility agent, which is first-line for the treatment of diarrhoea associated with irritable bowel syndrome (IBS)

18.11. A copper-chelating agent, which can be used for the treatment of Wilson's disease (WD)

18.12. A glucocorticoid, which is often given as a first-line therapeutic to induce remission in Crohn's disease (CD)

Theme

Disease-modifying anti-rheumatic drugs (DMARDs)

Options

- **A)** Azathioprine (AZA)
- **B)** Mesalazine (MSZ)
- **C)** Sulfasalazine (SSZ)
- **D)** Methotrexate (MTX)
- **E)** Infliximab (IFX)
- **F)** Rituximab (RTX)
- **G)** Tocilizumab (TZ)
- **H)** Hydroxychloroquine (HCQ)

Instructions

For each question in the list below (18.13.-18.18.), choose the single most appropriate answer from the list above (A-H). Each option may be used once, more than once or not at all.

Questions

18.13. An antimetabolite drug, which inhibits folic acid production by inhibiting the enzyme dihydrofolate reductase (DHFR)

18.14. An antimetabolite drug, which inhibits purine synthesis and subsequently interferes with deoxyribonucleic acid (DNA) and ribonucleic acid (RNA) production

18.15. An aminosalicylate anti-inflammatory agent, which is a well-established, first-line treatment for mild-to-moderate ulcerative colitis (UC)

18.16. A chimeric monoclonal antibody (mAb), which inhibits CD20-mediated B-cell differentiation and proliferation

18.17. A chimeric monoclonal antibody (mAb), which inhibits tumour necrosis factor alpha (TNF-α)

18.18. A monoclonal antibody (mAb), which is directed against the interleukin-6-receptor (IL-6)

Theme

Neuropharmacology

Options

- A) Pyridostigmine
- B) Lamotrigine
- C) Carbamazepine
- D) Sodium valproate
- E) Ropinirole
- F) Verapamil
- G) Propranolol
- H) Topiramate

Instructions

For each question in the list below (18.19.-18.24.), choose the single most appropriate answer from the list above (A-H). Each option may be used once, more than once or not at all.

Questions

18.19. A dopamine agonist, which is commonly used as a first-line therapy for younger patients with newly diagnosed Parkinson's disease (PD), in preference to initial treatment with levodopa (L-DOPA) and a peripheral decarboxylase inhibitor

18.20. An acetylcholinesterase (AChE) inhibitor, which is often given as a first-line treatment for myasthenia gravis (MG)

18.21. An anti-epileptic drug (AED), which inhibits glutamate release, stabilises inactive voltage-gated sodium channels and is a common first-line treatment for generalised seizures in women of childbearing age

18.22. An anti-epileptic drug (AED), which acts by inhibiting GABA transaminase (the enzyme primarily responsible for degradation of the inhibitory neurotransmitter, GABA) and serves as a first-line treatment for generalised seizures

18.23. An anti-epileptic drug (AED), which acts by stabilising inactive voltage-gated sodium channels, is a potent inducer of the cytochrome P450 enzyme system and serves as a first-line treatment for focal (partial) seizures

18.24. A β-blocker, which is commonly given for migraine prophylaxis

CHAPTER 18

Pharmacology and Therapeutics II (EMQs)

Answers and Detailed Solutions

The difficulty rating for each question (Easy, Moderate or Hard) can be found in parentheses next to the correct answer.

18.1. D (Hard)
18.2. A (Easy)
18.3. B (Moderate)
18.4. G (Hard)
18.5. H (Easy)
18.6. E (Easy)

The first-line drug in the emergency treatment of hyperkalaemia is intravenous (IV) calcium gluconate. This serves to protect the myocardium from the deleterious effects of high potassium levels. Following cardiac stabilisation, nebulised (neb) salbutamol is given, along with a dextrose and insulin infusion. This combination therapy serves to lower serum potassium levels by shifting potassium intracellularly. The potassium-binding agent, calcium resonium, is also given - orally or by enema - as it removes potassium from the body. Octreotide is a somatostatin analogue, used for the medical management of acromegaly, as it physiologically inhibits growth hormone (GH) secretion. The medical management of a phaeochromocytoma involves α-adrenergic blockade (phenoxybenzamine) followed by β-adrenergic blockade (propranolol). Amiodarone is an antiarrhythmic drug that can precipitate both hyperthyroidism and hypothyroidism. Carbimazole is a drug treatment for thyrotoxicosis, which can cause agranulocytosis (a low white blood cell count) in rare cases. Conversely, levothyroxine is a synthetic thyroid hormone used for the treatment of hypothyroidism.

18.7. B (Easy)
18.8. C (Easy)
18.9. A (Easy)
18.10. E (Moderate)
18.11. H (Hard)
18.12. G (Easy)

N-acetylcysteine (NAC) is the treatment of choice for acetaminophen (paracetamol) poisoning. Omeprazole and lansoprazole are both proton pump inhibitors (PPIs), which reduce gastric acid secretion by irreversibly inhibiting the hydrogen-potassium ATPase enzyme system in gastric parietal cells. Cinnarizine and cyclizine are antihistamines (H_1-receptor antagonists), which have antiemetic properties and can be used to treat Ménière's disease (a rare disorder characterised by vertigo, hearing loss and tinnitus). Ondansetron and granisetron are 5-hydroxytryptamine type 3 (5-HT_3) receptor antagonists, most commonly used for the prevention of chemotherapy-induced nausea and vomiting (N&V). Loperamide is an anti-motility agent, which is first-line for the treatment of diarrhoea associated with irritable bowel syndrome (IBS). Penicillamine is a copper-chelating agent, which can be used for the treatment of Wilson's disease (WD). Prednisolone is a glucocorticoid, which is often given as a first-line therapeutic to induce remission in Crohn's disease (CD). Terlipressin is a vasoactive agent, which can be used for the emergency management of bleeding oesophageal varices.

18.13. D (Moderate)
18.14. A (Moderate)
18.15. B (Moderate)
18.16. F (Hard)
18.17. E (Hard)
18.18. G (Hard)

Methotrexate (MTX) is an antimetabolite drug, which inhibits folic acid production by inhibiting the enzyme dihydrofolate reductase (DHFR). Azathioprine (AZA) is an antimetabolite drug, which inhibits purine synthesis and subsequently interferes with deoxyribonucleic acid (DNA) and ribonucleic acid (RNA) production. Mesalazine (MSZ) is an aminosalicylate anti-inflammatory agent, which is a well-established, first-line treatment for mild-to-moderate ulcerative colitis (UC). Sulfasalazine (SSZ) is a conjugate of mesalazine, which is widely used in combination with methotrexate and short-term glucocorticoids for the treatment of rheumatoid arthritis (RA). Infliximab (IFX) is a chimeric monoclonal antibody (mAb), which inhibits tumour necrosis factor alpha (TNF-α).

CHAPTER 18: Pharmacology and Therapeutics II (EMQs)

Likewise, rituximab (RTX) is a chimeric monoclonal antibody, which inhibits CD20-mediated B-cell differentiation and proliferation. Tocilizumab (TZ) is a monoclonal antibody, which is directed against the interleukin-6-receptor (IL-6). Finally, hydroxychloroquine (HCQ) is a commonly used disease-modifying anti-rheumatic drug (DMARD), which can cause retinal toxicity, classically producing a bull's eye maculopathy (BEM).

18.19. E (Hard)
18.20. A (Moderate)
18.21. B (Hard)
18.22. D (Moderate)
18.23. C (Moderate)
18.24. G (Easy)

Levodopa (L-DOPA) is the mainstay of therapy for the symptomatic treatment of Parkinson's disease (PD). This is given in combination with a peripheral decarboxylase inhibitor, to ensure that levodopa is not broken down by the enzyme dopa-decarboxylase in the periphery, before it crosses into the brain. The dopamine agonist, ropinirole, is commonly used as a first-line therapy for younger patients with newly diagnosed Parkinson's disease, in preference to initial treatment with levodopa and a peripheral decarboxylase inhibitor. This is because the effects of levodopa will wear off with time, and motor side effects can develop after 5-10 years of treatment with levodopa. Lamotrigine is an anti-epileptic drug (AED), which acts by inhibiting glutamate release and stabilising inactive voltage-gated sodium channels. This anticonvulsant is a common first-line treatment for generalised seizures in women of childbearing age, due to the teratogenic profile of sodium valproate. Carbamazepine is an anti-epileptic drug, which acts by stabilising inactive voltage-gated sodium channels, is a potent inducer of the cytochrome P450 enzyme system and serves as a first-line treatment for focal (partial) seizures. Sodium valproate is an anti-epileptic drug, which acts by inhibiting GABA transaminase (the enzyme primarily responsible for degradation of the inhibitory neurotransmitter, GABA) and serves as a first-line treatment for generalised seizures. The β-blocker, propranolol, is commonly given for migraine prophylaxis. The anti-epileptic drug, topiramate, can also be given for migraine prophylaxis, albeit not in women of childbearing age due to its teratogenic effects. Along similar lines, the calcium channel blocker (CCB), verapamil, is widely used for cluster headache prophylaxis. Pyridostigmine is an acetylcholinesterase (AChE) inhibitor, which is often given as a first-line treatment for myasthenia gravis (MG).

CHAPTER 19
Pharmacology and Therapeutics III (EMQs)

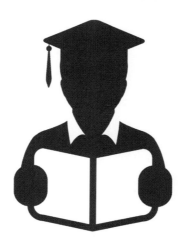

Theme

Antimicrobial agents

Options

A) Fluconazole
B) Flucloxacillin
C) Gentamicin
D) Vancomycin
E) Anidulafungin
F) Metronidazole
G) Trimethoprim
H) Caspofungin

Instructions

For each question in the list below (19.1.-19.6.), choose the single most appropriate answer from the list above (A-H). Each option may be used once, more than once or not at all.

Questions

19.1. Antibacterial cell wall synthesis inhibitor, with no gram-negative activity, which can cause nephrotoxicity and ototoxicity
19.2. Antibacterial protein synthesis inhibitor, with no activity against anaerobes, which can cause nephrotoxicity and ototoxicity
19.3. Antibacterial deoxyribonucleic acid (DNA) synthesis inhibitor, which is first-line in the treatment of uncomplicated urinary tract infections (UTIs)
19.4. Antibacterial cell wall synthesis inhibitor, which is the first-line treatment for uncomplicated cellulitis
19.5. A glycopeptide, which can cause diffuse flushing ("red person syndrome") if administered too quickly
19.6. A synthetic antibacterial and antiprotozoal agent, which is the first-line treatment for antibiotic-associated diarrhoea due to *Clostridium difficile (C. diff)* infection

Theme

The pharmacological management of tuberculosis (TB) and antibiotic therapy in lower respiratory tract infections (LRTIs)

Options

- A) Ethambutol
- B) Rifampicin
- C) Doxycycline
- D) Pyrazinamide
- E) Clarithromycin
- F) Isoniazid
- G) Co-trimoxazole
- H) Streptomycin

Instructions

For each question in the list below (19.7.-19.12.), choose the single most appropriate answer from the list above (A-H). Each option may be used once, more than once or not at all.

Questions

19.7. A bacterial ribonucleic acid (RNA) synthesis inhibitor, which is used to treat tuberculosis (TB), is a potent inducer of the cytochrome P450 enzyme system and can cause an orange-red discolouration of body secretions (tears, sweat and urine as well as other body fluids)

19.8. A chemotherapeutic agent, which is used to treat tuberculosis (TB) and is a known cause of optic neuropathy

19.9. A chemotherapeutic agent, which is used to treat tuberculosis (TB), is a relatively potent inhibitor of the cytochrome P450 enzyme system and is often co-administered with pyridoxine (vitamin B$_6$) in order to prevent peripheral neuropathy

19.10. A chemotherapeutic agent, which is used to treat tuberculosis (TB) and is associated with hepatotoxicity and gout (hyperuricaemia)

19.11. A macrolide, which can be given alongside amoxicillin to treat community-acquired pneumonia (CAP) if an atypical pathogen is suspected

19.12. An antibacterial deoxyribonucleic acid (DNA) synthesis inhibitor, which is also effective against the yeast-like fungus *pneumocystis jiroveci* (a cause of *Pneumocystis pneumonia* [PCP] in immunocompromised individuals)

CHAPTER 19: Pharmacology and Therapeutics III (EMQs)

Theme

Adverse drug reactions (ADRs)

Options

- A) Amiodarone
- B) Simvastatin
- C) Methotrexate (MTX)
- D) Isoniazid
- E) Propranolol
- F) Doxorubicin
- G) Sulfasalazine (SSZ)
- H) Hydralazine (HZ)

Instructions

For each question in the list below (19.13.-19.18.), choose the single most appropriate answer from the list above (A-H). Each option may be used once, more than once or not at all.

Questions

19.13. Deranged liver function tests (LFTs), myalgia, myositis and rhabdomyolysis (muscle breakdown)
19.14. Dilated cardiomyopathy (DCM)
19.15. Myelosuppression (bone marrow suppression), hepatic cirrhosis and pulmonary fibrosis
19.16. Bronchoconstriction in asthmatic patients
19.17. Slate-grey skin discolouration
19.18. Stevens-Johnson syndrome (SJS), pancreatitis, oligospermia and male infertility

Theme

Acute pain management

Options

- **A)** Morphine
- **B)** Pantoprazole
- **C)** Dihydrocodeine
- **D)** Paracetamol (acetaminophen)
- **E)** Ketamine
- **F)** Indomethacin
- **G)** Naloxone
- **H)** Gabapentin

Instructions

For each question in the list below (19.19.-19.24.), choose the single most appropriate answer from the list above (A-H). Each option may be used once, more than once or not at all.

Questions

19.19. A non-opioid analgesic, often used as an initial therapy for mild pain, which should never be given less than four hours apart

19.20. A non-steroidal anti-inflammatory drug (NSAID), often used for mild pain

19.21. A weak opioid analgesic, commonly given for mild to moderate pain

19.22. A strong opioid analgesic, commonly given for moderate to severe pain

19.23. An opioid antagonist, which is used for the treatment of opioid-induced respiratory depression

19.24. A proton pump inhibitor (PPI), often given alongside non-steroidal anti-inflammatory drugs (NSAIDs) to decrease the incidence of NSAID-related gastrointestinal (GI) side effects, such as ulceration, bleeding and perforation

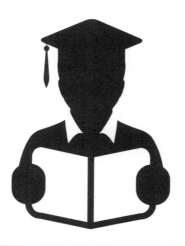

CHAPTER 19

Pharmacology and Therapeutics III (EMQs)

Answers and Detailed Solutions

The difficulty rating for each question (Easy, Moderate or Hard) can be found in parentheses next to the correct answer.

19.1. D (Moderate)
19.2. C (Moderate)
19.3. G (Easy)
19.4. B (Easy)
19.5. D (Moderate)
19.6. F (Moderate)

The glycopeptides, vancomycin and teicoplanin, are antibacterial cell wall synthesis inhibitors, with no gram-negative activity, which can cause nephrotoxicity and ototoxicity. Vancomycin can also cause diffuse flushing ("red person syndrome") if administered too quickly. The aminoglycosides, gentamicin and amikacin, are antibacterial protein synthesis inhibitors, with no activity against anaerobes, which can cause nephrotoxicity and ototoxicity. Flucloxacillin is an antibacterial cell wall synthesis inhibitor, which is the first-line treatment for uncomplicated cellulitis. Trimethoprim is an antibacterial deoxyribonucleic acid (DNA) synthesis inhibitor, which is first-line in the treatment of uncomplicated urinary tract infections (UTIs). Metronidazole is a synthetic antibacterial and antiprotozoal agent, which is the first-line treatment for antibiotic-associated diarrhoea due to *Clostridium difficile (C. diff)* infection. The echinocandins, anidulafungin and caspofungin, are antifungal cell wall synthesis inhibitors. The triazole antifungal, fluconazole, is a potent inhibitor of the cytochrome P450 enzyme system, which acts by inhibiting the synthesis of ergosterol, a component of the fungal cell membrane.

19.7. B (Hard)
19.8. A (Hard)
19.9. F (Hard)
19.10. D (Hard)
19.11. E (Moderate)
19.12. G (Hard)

Rifampicin, isoniazid, pyrazinamide, ethambutol and streptomycin are all used in the pharmacological management of tuberculosis (TB). Rifampicin is a bacterial ribonucleic acid (RNA) synthesis inhibitor, which can cause an orange-red discolouration of body secretions (tears, sweat and urine as well as other body fluids) and it is also a potent inducer of the cytochrome P450 enzyme system. Isoniazid is a chemotherapeutic agent, which is often co-administered with pyridoxine (vitamin B_6) in order to prevent peripheral neuropathy and it is also a relatively potent inhibitor of the cytochrome P450 enzyme system. Ethambutol is a chemotherapeutic agent and a known cause of optic neuropathy. Likewise, pyrazinamide is a chemotherapeutic agent, which is associated with hepatotoxicity and gout (hyperuricaemia). The aminoglycoside, streptomycin, is also a chemotherapeutic agent, which acts by inhibiting bacterial protein synthesis. Co-trimoxazole is an antibacterial deoxyribonucleic acid (DNA) synthesis inhibitor, which is also effective against the yeast-like fungus *pneumocystis jiroveci* (a cause of *Pneumocystis pneumonia* [PCP] in immunocompromised individuals). Clarithromycin is a macrolide, which can be given alongside amoxicillin to treat community-acquired pneumonia (CAP) if an atypical pathogen is suspected. Similarly, doxycycline is a tetracycline, which can be given as a monotherapy for moderate-severity community-acquired pneumonia.

19.13. B (Easy)
19.14. F (Hard)
19.15. C (Moderate)
19.16. E (Easy)
19.17. A (Hard)
19.18. G (Hard)

Beta blockers, such as propranolol, are often contraindicated in asthmatic patients, as they can cause bronchoconstriction. The disease-modifying anti-rheumatic drug (DMARD), sulfasalazine (SSZ), can precipitate Stevens-Johnson syndrome (SJS), pancreatitis, oligospermia and male infertility. The anthracycline anticancer agent, doxorubicin, is a known cause of dilated cardiomyopathy (DCM). Statins, such as simvastatin, can cause deranged liver function tests (LFTs), myalgia, myositis and rhabdomyolysis (muscle breakdown). The antimetabolite drug, methotrexate (MTX), can precipitate myelosuppression (bone marrow suppression), hepatic cirrhosis and pulmonary fibrosis. The antiarrhythmic drug, amiodarone, can produce a characteristic slate-grey skin discolouration. Hydralazine (HZ) and isoniazid are both associated with a high incidence of drug-induced lupus erythematosus (DILE), as are other drugs, such as procainamide, minocycline and penicillamine.

19.19. D (Easy)
19.20. F (Moderate)
19.21. C (Easy)
19.22. A (Easy)
19.23. G (Moderate)
19.24. B (Easy)

Paracetamol (acetaminophen) is a non-opioid analgesic, often used as an initial therapy for mild pain, which should never be given less than four hours apart. If mild pain persists following the administration of paracetamol, a non-steroidal anti-inflammatory drug (NSAID), such as indomethacin, can also be given. Proton pump inhibitors (PPIs), such as pantoprazole, are commonly given alongside non-steroidal anti-inflammatory drugs (NSAIDs) in order to decrease the incidence of NSAID-related gastrointestinal (GI) side effects, such as ulceration, bleeding and perforation. Dihydrocodeine is a weak opioid analgesic, given for mild to moderate pain, while morphine is a strong opioid analgesic, routinely given for moderate to severe pain. Naloxone is an opioid antagonist, which is used for the treatment of opioid-induced respiratory depression. The anticonvulsant, gabapentin, and the N-methyl-D-aspartate (NMDA) receptor antagonist, ketamine, are both non-opioid-based adjuvant analgesic agents.

CHAPTER 20
Clinical Biochemistry (EMQs)

Theme

Autoantibodies as a diagnostic tool for specific rheumatic diseases

Options

A) Rheumatoid arthritis (RA)
B) Mixed connective tissue disease (MCTD)
C) Systemic lupus erythematosus (SLE)
D) Drug-induced lupus erythematosus (DILE)
E) Sjogren's syndrome (SS)
F) Diffuse cutaneous systemic sclerosis (dcSSc)
G) Limited cutaneous systemic sclerosis (lcSSc)
H) Dermatomyositis (DM) and polymyositis (PM)

Instructions

For each question in the list below (20.1.-20.6.), choose the single most appropriate answer from the list above (A-H). Each option may be used once, more than once or not at all.

Questions

20.1. Antinuclear antibody (ANA), anti-double stranded DNA antibody (anti-dsDNA) and anti-Smith (anti-Sm) antibodies
20.2. Rheumatoid factor (RF) and anti-cyclic citrullinated peptide (anti-CCP) antibodies
20.3. Anti-Ro (SSA) antibodies and anti-La (SSB) antibodies
20.4. Anti-histone antibodies (AHA)
20.5. Anti-centromere antibodies (ACA)
20.6. Anti-topoisomerase I (Scl-70) antibodies

Theme

Hepatotropic viruses and hepatitis B serology

Options

- **A)** Antibody to hepatitis B core antigen (anti-HBc)
- **B)** Antibody to hepatitis B e antigen (anti-HBe)
- **C)** Antibody to hepatitis B surface antigen (anti-HBs)
- **D)** Hepatitis A virus (HAV)
- **E)** Hepatitis B e antigen (HBeAg)
- **F)** Hepatitis B surface antigen (HBsAg)
- **G)** Hepatitis D virus (HDV)
- **H)** Hepatitis E virus (HEV)

Instructions

For each question in the list below (20.7.-20.12.), choose the single most appropriate answer from the list above (A-H). Each option may be used once, more than once or not at all.

Questions

20.7. The first serological marker to appear in hepatitis B virus (HBV) infection, which is present in acute or chronic (if present for more than 6 months) HBV infection

20.8. The only serological marker detectable after immunisation with the HBV vaccine

20.9. Commonly used as an index of infectivity, and correlates with HBV replication and high infectivity

20.10. Indicates past or current HBV infection, and is found in immunity that is naturally acquired (not vaccine-induced immunity)

20.11. A single stranded ribonucleic acid (RNA) virus, which has a particular morbidity in pregnant women

20.12. Infection occurs simultaneously with HBV infection or as a superinfection in patients already infected with HBV

CHAPTER 20: Clinical Biochemistry (EMQs)

Theme

Serum biochemistry in metabolic bone disease (MBD)

Options

Metabolic bone disease (MBD)	Calcium (Ca)	Phosphate	Alkaline phosphatase (ALP)	Parathyroid hormone (PTH)
A	↑	↓	↑	↑
B	↑	↑	↑	↑
C	⇔	⇔	⇔	⇔
D	⇔	⇔	↑	⇔
E	↓	↓	↑	↑
F	↓	↑	⇔	↓
G	↑	⇔	⇔	⇔
H	↓	↑	↑	↑

* ⇔ = Normal   ↑ = Increased   ↓ = Decreased

Instructions

For each question in the list below (20.13.-20.18.), choose the single most appropriate answer from the table above (A-H). Each option may be used once, more than once or not at all.

Questions

20.13. Osteoporosis
20.14. Osteomalacia
20.15. Paget's disease (PD)
20.16. Primary hyperparathyroidism (pHPT)
20.17. Secondary hyperparathyroidism (sHPT)
20.18. Tertiary hyperparathyroidism (tHPT)

Theme

Red blood cell (RBC) morphology and important clinical associations

Options

- **A)** Basophilic stippling (punctate basophilia)
- **B)** Howell-Jolly bodies (HJB)
- **C)** Hypersegmented neutrophils (HN)
- **D)** Spherocytes
- **E)** 'Tear-drop' poikilocytes (dacrocytes)
- **F)** Heinz bodies (Heinz-Ehrlich bodies)
- **G)** Schistocytes (helmet cells)
- **H)** 'Pencil' poikilocytes

Instructions

For each question in the list below (20.19.-20.24.), choose the single most appropriate answer from the list above (A-H). Each option may be used once, more than once or not at all.

Questions

20.19. Hyposplenism, post-splenectomy and megaloblastic anaemia (MBA)

20.20. Lead poisoning (LP), pyrimidine-5'-nucleotidase (P5N) deficiency, thalassaemia, myelodysplastic syndromes (MDS, or myelodysplasia) and sideroblastic anaemia (SA)

20.21. Autoimmune haemolytic anaemia (AIHA) and hereditary spherocytosis (HS)

20.22. Myelofibrosis (MF)

20.23. Glucose-6-phosphate dehydrogenase (GP6D) deficiency

20.24. Intravascular haemolysis (IVH), thrombotic thrombocytopenic purpura (TTP), disseminated intravascular coagulation (DIC), malignant hypertension and artificial heart valves (AHV)

CHAPTER 20

Clinical Biochemistry (EMQs)

Answers and Detailed Solutions

The difficulty rating for each question (Easy, Moderate or Hard) can be found in parentheses next to the correct answer.

20.1. C (Moderate)
20.2. A (Easy)
20.3. E (Hard)
20.4. D (Hard)
20.5. G (Hard)
20.6. F (Hard)

The following table highlights the autoantibodies characteristically associated with specific rheumatic diseases:

Rheumatic Disease	Autoantibodies
Rheumatoid arthritis (RA)	Rheumatoid factor (RF) and anti-cyclic citrullinated peptide (anti-CCP) antibodies
Mixed connective tissue disease (MCTD)	Anti-RNP antibodies
Systemic lupus erythematosus (SLE)	Antinuclear antibody (ANA), anti-double stranded DNA antibody (anti-dsDNA) and anti-Smith (anti-Sm) antibodies
Drug-induced lupus erythematosus (DILE)	Anti-histone antibodies (AHA)
Sjogren's syndrome (SS)	Anti-Ro (SSA) antibodies and anti-La (SSB) antibodies
Diffuse cutaneous systemic sclerosis (dcSSc)	Anti-topoisomerase I (Scl-70) antibodies
Limited cutaneous systemic sclerosis (lcSSc)	Anti-centromere antibodies (ACA)
Dermatomyositis (DM) and polymyositis (PM)	Anti-Jo-1 antibodies

[This table is by no means exhaustive, rather it lists the autoantibodies most commonly associated with specific rheumatic diseases.]

20.7. F (Moderate)
20.8. C (Hard)
20.9. E (Moderate)
20.10. A (Hard)
20.11. H (Easy)
20.12. G (Easy)

Hepatitis A virus (HAV) is a single stranded ribonucleic acid (RNA) virus, which is transmitted via the faecal-oral route and is associated with the consumption of raw or poorly cooked shellfish. Hepatitis D virus (HDV) is a defective single stranded ribonucleic acid virus that cannot cause disease on its own. As such, infection occurs simultaneously with hepatitis B virus (HBV) infection or as a superinfection in patients already infected with HBV. Hepatitis E virus (HEV) is a single stranded ribonucleic acid virus, which has a particular morbidity in pregnant women. Hepatitis B surface antigen (HBsAg) is the first serological marker to appear in hepatitis B virus infection, and it is present in acute or chronic (if present for more than 6 months) HBV infection. Antibody to hepatitis B surface antigen (anti-HBs) is the only serological marker detectable after immunisation with the HBV vaccine. In contrast, antibody to hepatitis B core antigen (anti-HBc) indicates past or current HBV infection, and is found in immunity that is naturally acquired (not vaccine-induced immunity). Hepatitis B e antigen (HBeAg) is commonly used as an index of infectivity, and correlates with HBV replication and high infectivity, while antibody to hepatitis B e antigen (anti-HBe) correlates with low HBV replication and low infectivity.

20.13. C (Easy)
20.14. E (Easy)
20.15. D (Moderate)
20.16. A (Easy)
20.17. H (Easy)
20.18. B (Easy)

CHAPTER 20: Clinical Biochemistry (EMQs)

The following table highlights the typical serum biochemistry in different metabolic bone diseases (MBDs):

Metabolic bone disease (MBD)	Calcium (Ca)	Phosphate	Alkaline phosphatase (ALP)	Parathyroid hormone (PTH)
Primary hyperparathyroidism (pHPT)	↑	↓	↑	↑
Secondary hyperparathyroidism (sHPT)	↓	↑	↑	↑
Tertiary hyperparathyroidism (tHPT)	↑	↑	↑	↑
Osteoporosis	⇔	⇔	⇔	⇔
Paget's disease (PD)	⇔	⇔	↑	⇔
Osteomalacia	↓	↓	↑	↑
Hypoparathyroidism	↓	↑	⇔	↓
Multiple myeloma (MM)	↑	⇔	⇔	⇔

* ⇔ = Normal   ↑ = Increased   ↓ = Decreased

For further information about osteoporosis, osteomalacia, Paget's disease, primary hyperparathyroidism, secondary hyperparathyroidism and tertiary hyperparathyroidism, refer to the detailed solutions for question 11.22. in chapter 11 and question 14.20. in chapter 14.

20.19. B (Moderate)
20.20. A (Moderate)
20.21. D (Moderate)
20.22. E (Hard)
20.23. F (Hard)
20.24. G (Moderate)

The following table highlights characteristic red blood cell (RBC) morphologies along with important clinical associations:

Red blood cell (RBC) morphology	Clinical associations
Basophilic stippling (punctate basophilia)	Lead poisoning (LP), pyrimidine-5'- nucleotidase (P5N) deficiency, thalassaemia, myelodysplastic syndromes (MDS, or myelodysplasia) and sideroblastic anaemia (SA)
Howell-Jolly bodies (HJB)	Hyposplenism, post-splenectomy and megaloblastic anaemia (MBA)
Heinz bodies (Heinz-Ehrlich bodies)	Glucose-6-phosphate dehydrogenase (GP6D) deficiency
Hypersegmented neutrophils (HN)	Megaloblastic anaemia (MBA)
'Pencil' poikilocytes	Iron deficiency anaemia (IDA)
Target cells (codocytes)	Liver disease (especially obstructive jaundice), iron deficiency anaemia (IDA), sickle cell disease (SCD), thalassaemia, post-splenectomy and hyposplenism
'Tear-drop' poikilocytes (dacrocytes)	Myelofibrosis (MF)
Spherocytes	Autoimmune haemolytic anaemia (AIHA) and hereditary spherocytosis (HS)
Schistocytes (helmet cells)	Intravascular haemolysis (IVH), thrombotic thrombocytopenic purpura (TTP), disseminated intravascular coagulation (DIC), malignant hypertension and artificial heart valves (AHV)

CHAPTER 21
Clinical Interpretation (EMQs)

Theme

Electrocardiogram (ECG) interpretation

Options

- **A)** Atrial fibrillation (AF)
- **B)** Atrial flutter (AFL)
- **C)** Hypokalaemia
- **D)** Hyperkalaemia
- **E)** Hypothermia
- **F)** Wolff-Parkinson-White (WPW) syndrome
- **G)** First-degree atrioventricular block (AV block)
- **H)** Third-degree atrioventricular block (AV block) or complete heart block (CHB)

Instructions

For each question in the list below (21.1.-21.6.), choose the single most appropriate answer from the list above (A-H). Each option may be used once, more than once or not at all.

Questions

- **21.1.** Prominent U waves
- **21.2.** Prominent J waves
- **21.3.** No P waves and an irregularly irregular rhythm
- **21.4.** Short PR interval with delta waves (slurred upstroke of the QRS complex)
- **21.5.** Sawtooth, undulating baseline and a regular rhythm
- **21.6.** Normal sinus rhythm, with a prolonged PR interval, caused by abnormally slow conduction through the atrioventricular (AV) node

Theme

Heart sounds and murmurs

Options

- **A)** Aortic stenosis (AS)
- **B)** Aortic regurgitation (AR)
- **C)** First heart sound (S_1)
- **D)** Mitral stenosis (MS)
- **E)** Mitral regurgitation (MR)
- **F)** Pulmonary stenosis (PS)
- **G)** Second heart sound (S_2)
- **H)** Tricuspid regurgitation (TR)

Instructions

For each question in the list below (21.7.-21.12.), choose the single most appropriate answer from the list above (A-H). Each option may be used once, more than once or not at all.

Questions

21.7. Early diastolic, high-pitched murmur, and a collapsing (water-hammer) pulse with a wide pulse pressure

21.8. Ejection systolic murmur (ESM), and a slow rising pulse with a narrow pulse pressure

21.9. A high-pitched, blowing pansystolic or holosystolic murmur, which often radiates to the axilla

21.10. A low-pitched, rumbling mid-diastolic murmur, often accompanied by an opening snap

21.11. Produced by closure of the aortic and pulmonary valves

21.12. A pansystolic or holosystolic murmur, and an elevated jugular venous pressure (JVP) with a prominent 'v' wave followed by a sharp 'y' descent

CHAPTER 21: Clinical Interpretation (EMQs)

Theme

Common orthopaedic fractures

Options

- A) Bennett's fracture
- B) Boxer's fracture
- C) Colles' fracture
- D) Galeazzi fracture
- E) Intertrochanteric hip fracture
- F) Scaphoid fracture
- G) Smith's fracture
- H) Subcapital hip fracture

Instructions

For each question in the list below (21.13.-21.18.), choose the single most appropriate answer from the list above (A-H). Each option may be used once, more than once or not at all.

Questions

21.13. A fracture of the distal radius with dorsal angulation of the distal fragment, which typically occurs in elderly, osteoporotic patients following a fall on an outstretched hand (FOOSH)

21.14. A fracture of the distal radius with volar (palmar) angulation of the distal fragment, commonly caused by falling onto a flexed wrist

21.15. A radial shaft fracture with dislocation or subluxation of the distal radio-ulnar joint (DRUJ)

21.16. An intracapsular hip fracture

21.17. An extracapsular hip fracture

21.18. Wrist pain following a fall on an outstretched hand (FOOSH), along with swelling and tenderness in the anatomical snuffbox on clinical examination

Theme

Cranial nerve (CN) lesions

Options

- **A)** CN III (the oculomotor nerve)
- **B)** CN IV (the trochlear nerve)
- **C)** CN VI (the abducens nerve)
- **D)** CN VII (the facial nerve)
- **E)** CN VIII (the vestibulocochlear nerve)
- **F)** CN X (the vagus nerve)
- **G)** CN XI (the accessory nerve)
- **H)** CN XII (the hypoglossal nerve)

Instructions

For each question in the list below (21.19.-21.24.), choose the single most appropriate answer from the list above (A-H). Each option may be used once, more than once or not at all.

Questions

- **21.19.** Horizontal diplopia (double vision) and an inability to abduct the affected eye past the midline
- **21.20.** Vertical diplopia and an inability to look 'down and in'
- **21.21.** Complete ptosis and an eye that is positioned 'down and out'
- **21.22.** Tongue deviates towards the side of the lesion
- **21.23.** Hearing loss, nystagmus, tinnitus and vertigo
- **21.24.** Weakness turning head towards contralateral side of the lesion and shoulder droop on the side of the lesion

CHAPTER 21

Clinical Interpretation (EMQs)

Answers and Detailed Solutions

The difficulty rating for each question (Easy, Moderate or Hard) can be found in parentheses next to the correct answer.

21.1. C (Hard)
21.2. E (Hard)
21.3. A (Moderate)
21.4. F (Hard)
21.5. B (Moderate)
21.6. G (Hard)

Atrial fibrillation (AF) and atrial flutter (AFL) are the first and second most common atrial tachyarrhythmias respectively. The former is marked by no P waves and a rapid, irregularly irregular rhythm while the latter is distinguished by a sawtooth, undulating baseline and a regular rhythm. Wolff-Parkinson-White (WPW) syndrome is characterised by a short PR interval with delta waves (slurred upstroke of the QRS complex), caused by a congenital accessory pathway that provides abnormal electrical communication between the atria and the ventricles. Prominent U waves are a typical ECG sign of hypokalaemia, while the development of prominent J waves is associated with hypothermia. Tall, peaked and symmetrical ('tented') T waves are the earliest ECG abnormality seen in hyperkalaemia, followed by flattened P waves, widened QRS complexes and a prolonged PR interval. First-degree atrioventricular block (AV block) is caused by abnormally slow conduction through the atrioventricular (AV) node, and is characterised by normal sinus rhythm, with a prolonged PR interval. In contrast, third-degree atrioventricular block or complete heart block (CHB) represents a complete failure of conduction through the atrioventricular node, and is thus characterised by regular P waves and regular QRS complexes, which are unrelated to each other.

21.7. B (Moderate)
21.8. A (Moderate)
21.9. E (Hard)
21.10. D (Hard)
21.11. G (Easy)
21.12. H (Hard)

The first heart sound (S$_1$) is associated with closure of the mitral and tricuspid valves ("lub"), while the second heart sound (S$_2$) is produced by closure of the aortic and pulmonary valves ("dub"). Aortic stenosis (AS) causes an ejection systolic murmur (ESM), and a slow rising pulse with a narrow pulse pressure. Conversely, aortic regurgitation (AR) produces an early diastolic, high-pitched murmur, and a collapsing (water-hammer) pulse with a wide pulse pressure. The murmur of mitral regurgitation (MR) is a high-pitched, blowing pansystolic or holosystolic murmur, which often radiates to the axilla. In contrast, the murmur of mitral stenosis (MS) is a low-pitched, rumbling mid-diastolic murmur, often accompanied by an opening snap. Tricuspid regurgitation (TR) is usually associated with a pansystolic or holosystolic murmur, and an elevated jugular venous pressure (JVP) with a prominent 'v' wave followed by a sharp 'y' descent. Pulmonary stenosis (PS) is characterised by an ejection systolic murmur and a prominent 'a' wave in the JVP.

21.13. C (Easy)
21.14. G (Easy)
21.15. D (Hard)
21.16. H (Easy)
21.17. E (Easy)
21.18. F (Moderate)

Hip fractures can be classified as either intracapsular (subcapital) or extracapsular (intertrochanteric). There is a risk of avascular necrosis (AVN) with the former, however, as the blood supply to the femoral head can be disrupted. The most common thumb fracture is a Bennett's fracture, which describes an intra-articular fracture of the base of the first metacarpal, along with dislocation of the carpometacarpal (CMC) joint. A boxer's fracture is the most common metacarpal fracture. This fifth metacarpal neck fracture is commonly caused by striking a solid object with a clenched fist. A scaphoid fracture should be clinically suspected when a patient presents with wrist pain following a fall on an outstretched hand (FOOSH), along with swelling and tenderness in the anatomical snuffbox on clinical examination. A Colles' fracture is a fracture of the distal radius with dorsal angulation of the distal fragment, which typically occurs in elderly, osteoporotic patients following a fall on an outstretched hand. Similarly, a Smith's fracture, otherwise known as a reverse Colles' fracture, is a fracture of the distal radius with volar (palmar) angulation of the distal fragment, commonly caused by falling onto a flexed wrist. A Galeazzi fracture is a radial shaft fracture with dislocation or subluxation of the distal radio-ulnar joint (DRUJ).

21.19. C (Moderate)
21.20. B (Moderate)
21.21. A (Moderate)
21.22. H (Easy)
21.23. E (Easy)
21.24. G (Easy)

Damage to the oculomotor nerve (CN III) can result in complete ptosis and an eye that is positioned 'down and out'. Vertical diplopia (double vision) and an inability to look 'down and in' are characteristic of a trochlear nerve (CN IV) palsy, while horizontal diplopia and an inability to abduct the affected eye past the midline can occur in an abducens nerve (CN VI) palsy. Damage to the facial nerve (CN VII) can result in paralysis of the muscles of facial expression, hyperacusis (auditory hyperesthesia) and a loss of taste over the ipsilateral anterior 2/3^{rds} of the tongue. Similarly, hearing loss, nystagmus, tinnitus and vertigo can all be seen following injury to the vestibulocochlear nerve (CN VIII). Lesions of the vagus nerve (CN X) can cause deviation of the uvula away from the side of damage. Patients with an accessory nerve (CN XI) lesion will often exhibit weakness when turning their head towards the contralateral side of the lesion, as well as shoulder droop on the side of the lesion. Likewise, a lesion of the hypoglossal nerve (CN XII) will cause the tongue to deviate towards the side of the lesion. For further information about the location and function of each of the twelve cranial nerves, refer to the detailed solutions for questions 15.9., 15.10., 15.11., 15.12. and 15.13. in chapter 15.

ANSWER KEY

Chapter 1: Cell and Tissue Biology

Question	Answer
1.1	C
1.2	C
1.3	D
1.4	C
1.5	A
1.6	C
1.7	D
1.8	B
1.9	A
1.10	B
1.11	A
1.12	D
1.13	B
1.14	C
1.15	C
1.16	A
1.17	B
1.18	A
1.19	C
1.20	B
1.21	B
1.22	D
1.23	D
1.24	B

Chapter 2: Proteins

Question	Answer
2.1	C
2.2	A
2.3	B
2.4	B
2.5	B
2.6	A
2.7	C
2.8	C
2.9	A
2.10	C
2.11	D
2.12	A
2.13	A
2.14	A
2.15	A
2.16	D
2.17	C
2.18	B
2.19	B
2.20	B
2.21	B
2.22	A
2.23	B
2.24	B

Chapter 3: Enzymes and Metabolism

Question	Answer
3.1	B
3.2	D
3.3	B
3.4	A
3.5	B
3.6	A
3.7	C
3.8	B
3.9	C
3.10	D
3.11	C
3.12	D
3.13	C
3.14	D
3.15	D
3.16	D
3.17	A
3.18	B
3.19	D
3.20	B
3.21	A
3.22	C
3.23	D
3.24	D

Chapter 4: Clinical Genetics

Question	Answer
4.1	C
4.2	D
4.3	A
4.4	A
4.5	D
4.6	B
4.7	D
4.8	D
4.9	B
4.10	A
4.11	A
4.12	B
4.13	B
4.14	B
4.15	C
4.16	C
4.17	B
4.18	C
4.19	D
4.20	B
4.21	D
4.22	A
4.23	B
4.24	B

Answer Key

Chapter 5: Embryology and Reproduction

Question	Answer
5.1	C
5.2	B
5.3	B
5.4	B
5.5	D
5.6	C
5.7	D
5.8	A
5.9	B
5.10	C
5.11	A
5.12	C
5.13	B
5.14	D
5.15	D
5.16	D
5.17	C
5.18	D
5.19	D
5.20	A
5.21	C
5.22	A
5.23	A
5.24	D

Chapter 6: The Respiratory System

Question	Answer
6.1	B
6.2	C
6.3	B
6.4	B
6.5	B
6.6	A
6.7	B
6.8	D
6.9	B
6.10	B
6.11	A
6.12	C
6.13	B
6.14	A
6.15	C
6.16	B
6.17	A
6.18	A
6.19	C
6.20	D
6.21	B
6.22	D
6.23	C
6.24	A

Chapter 7: The Cardiovascular System

Question	Answer
7.1	A
7.2	C
7.3	C
7.4	B
7.5	A
7.6	B
7.7	C
7.8	B
7.9	B
7.10	D
7.11	A
7.12	A
7.13	D
7.14	A
7.15	C
7.16	B
7.17	D
7.18	C
7.19	D
7.20	D
7.21	D
7.22	A
7.23	C
7.24	C

Chapter 8: The Gastrointestinal System

Question	Answer
8.1	B
8.2	D
8.3	B
8.4	C
8.5	B
8.6	A
8.7	C
8.8	B
8.9	D
8.10	C
8.11	B
8.12	A
8.13	C
8.14	C
8.15	C
8.16	A
8.17	C
8.18	B
8.19	C
8.20	D
8.21	D
8.22	C
8.23	B
8.24	A

Answer Key

Chapter 9: The Renal System

Question	Answer
9.1	D
9.2	B
9.3	D
9.4	C
9.5	D
9.6	D
9.7	C
9.8	D
9.9	B
9.10	C
9.11	A
9.12	B
9.13	B
9.14	C
9.15	A
9.16	C
9.17	A
9.18	C
9.19	A
9.20	C
9.21	D
9.22	A
9.23	D
9.24	A

Chapter 10: Haematology

Question	Answer
10.1	B
10.2	C
10.3	C
10.4	D
10.5	B
10.6	A
10.7	D
10.8	A
10.9	C
10.10	C
10.11	C
10.12	A
10.13	B
10.14	A
10.15	B
10.16	D
10.17	A
10.18	B
10.19	C
10.20	C
10.21	B
10.22	B
10.23	A
10.24	B

Chapter 11: Endocrinology

Question	Answer
11.1	B
11.2	C
11.3	A
11.4	B
11.5	D
11.6	B
11.7	C
11.8	A
11.9	D
11.10	D
11.11	A
11.12	D
11.13	C
11.14	C
11.15	C
11.16	D
11.17	A
11.18	C
11.19	D
11.20	B
11.21	D
11.22	B
11.23	C
11.24	B

Chapter 12: The Immune System

Question	Answer
12.1	D
12.2	C
12.3	D
12.4	C
12.5	C
12.6	B
12.7	D
12.8	A
12.9	B
12.10	D
12.11	B
12.12	A
12.13	C
12.14	A
12.15	B
12.16	A
12.17	D
12.18	B
12.19	A
12.20	A
12.21	D
12.22	C
12.23	B
12.24	A

Answer Key

Chapter 13: Microbiology and Infection

Question	Answer
13.1	C
13.2	B
13.3	B
13.4	B
13.5	A
13.6	D
13.7	B
13.8	A
13.9	D
13.10	C
13.11	A
13.12	B
13.13	D
13.14	B
13.15	B
13.16	C
13.17	A
13.18	A
13.19	A
13.20	A
13.21	B
13.22	D
13.23	D
13.24	C

Chapter 14: The Musculoskeletal System

Question	Answer
14.1	C
14.2	B
14.3	B
14.4	A
14.5	C
14.6	C
14.7	B
14.8	D
14.9	A
14.10	B
14.11	A
14.12	D
14.13	A
14.14	C
14.15	D
14.16	C
14.17	C
14.18	B
14.19	C
14.20	C
14.21	C
14.22	A
14.23	C
14.24	D

Chapter 15: The Nervous System

Question	Answer
15.1	C
15.2	D
15.3	C
15.4	D
15.5	B
15.6	B
15.7	D
15.8	D
15.9	B
15.10	B
15.11	D
15.12	D
15.13	B
15.14	D
15.15	B
15.16	D
15.17	C
15.18	C
15.19	C
15.20	C
15.21	C
15.22	C
15.23	A
15.24	C

Chapter 16: Public Health

Question	Answer
16.1	F
16.2	A
16.3	E
16.4	G
16.5	C
16.6	D
16.7	E
16.8	D
16.9	A
16.10	C
16.11	H
16.12	G
16.13	A
16.14	G
16.15	H
16.16	B
16.17	D
16.18	E
16.19	A
16.20	C
16.21	E
16.22	H
16.23	D
16.24	F

Answer Key

Chapter 17: Pharmacology and Therapeutics I

Question	Answer
17.1	G
17.2	E
17.3	H
17.4	F
17.5	C
17.6	D
17.7	C
17.8	D
17.9	F
17.10	H
17.11	B
17.12	G
17.13	B
17.14	F
17.15	D
17.16	A
17.17	E
17.18	C
17.19	C
17.20	A
17.21	B
17.22	D
17.23	G
17.24	E

Chapter 18: Pharmacology and Therapeutics II

Question	Answer
18.1	D
18.2	A
18.3	B
18.4	G
18.5	H
18.6	E
18.7	B
18.8	C
18.9	A
18.10	E
18.11	H
18.12	G
18.13	D
18.14	A
18.15	B
18.16	F
18.17	E
18.18	G
18.19	E
18.20	A
18.21	B
18.22	D
18.23	C
18.24	G

Chapter 19: Pharmacology and Therapeutics III

Question	Answer
19.1	D
19.2	C
19.3	G
19.4	B
19.5	D
19.6	F
19.7	B
19.8	A
19.9	F
19.10	D
19.11	E
19.12	G
19.13	B
19.14	F
19.15	C
19.16	E
19.17	A
19.18	G
19.19	D
19.20	F
19.21	C
19.22	A
19.23	G
19.24	B

Chapter 20: Clinical Biochemistry

Question	Answer
20.1	C
20.2	A
20.3	E
20.4	D
20.5	G
20.6	F
20.7	F
20.8	C
20.9	E
20.10	A
20.11	H
20.12	G
20.13	C
20.14	E
20.15	D
20.16	A
20.17	H
20.18	B
20.19	B
20.20	A
20.21	D
20.22	E
20.23	F
20.24	G

Chapter 21:
Clinical Interpretation

Question	Answer
21.1	C
21.2	E
21.3	A
21.4	F
21.5	B
21.6	G
21.7	B
21.8	A
21.9	E
21.10	D
21.11	G
21.12	H
21.13	C
21.14	G
21.15	D
21.16	H
21.17	E
21.18	F
21.19	C
21.20	B
21.21	A
21.22	H
21.23	E
21.24	G

Confirmed Future Titles in the *With Honours* Series

GAMSAT Written Communication: A Practical Guide to Essay Composition

GAMSAT Chemistry: Practice Questions with Detailed Solutions

GAMSAT Physics: Practice Questions with Detailed Solutions

MCAT Biology: Practice Questions with Detailed Solutions

SAT Subject Test Italian: Practice Questions with Detailed Solutions

GCSE (9-1) French: Practice Questions with Detailed Solutions

For further information about the *With Honours* series and any other enquiries, please visit us at withhonours.co.uk or send us an email at: contact@withhonours.co.uk

 Facebook @WithHonours

 Twitter @With_Honours

 Pinterest with_honours

 Instagram @with_honours

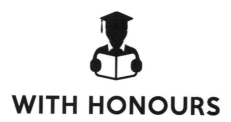

WITH HONOURS

Printed in Great Britain
by Amazon